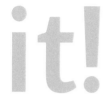

D1706426

Reverse

The 40-day plan of words and recipes to jumpstart the reversal of type 2 diabetes and other chronic diseases

Because you can!

Printed in the United States of America First Printing December 2018

Important Legal Notice and Disclaimer

Neither Pain 2 Wellness Healthcare, the publisher nor the author is engaged in rendering professional advice or services to the individual reader. The ideas, procedures and suggestions in this book are not intended as a substitute for sound medical advice from your rendering physician. All matters of health require medical supervision. Neither the author nor the publisher shall be liable or responsible for any loss or damage allegedly arising from any information or suggestion in this book.

The recipes in this book are to be followed as written. Pain 2 Wellness Healthcare, nor the publisher nor the author is responsible for specific health or allergy needs that may require medical supervision or for any adverse reactions to these recipes.

While the author has made every effort to provide accurate citation information that may include internet information at the time of publication, neither Pain 2 Wellness Healthcare, the publisher nor the author assumes any responsibility for errors, or for changes that occur after publication. Further, the publisher does not have any control over and does not assume any responsibility for the author or third-party websites or their content.

"This book by Dr. Powell-Stoddart is not covering a new treatment approach. That treatment has been documented as being most effective in reversing Type 2 diabetes since 1927. What is new is that she has put together a very doable 40-day dietary plan of "foods-as-grown" that helps to jumpstart the reversal process in a consistent manner, activating the body's self-healing mechanisms, and leading comfortably right into the adaptability of the Whole Food Plant-based diet. In the process another vital discovery can be made—we as consumers are the CEOs of our own health. We must take action. This plan enables the reader to do just that!"

—HANS DIEHL DrHSC, MPH
Clinical Professor of Preventive Medicine
School of Medicine, Loma Linda University
Founder: Lifestyle Medicine Institute & CHIP

In this book, Dr. Powell-Stoddart shares a very touching personal story of tragic losses that we can all relate to. Through her experience she learns about the power of plant-based diets, and begins transforming lives. **Reverse It!** provides a solid 40-day program to jumpstart your journey to health using a highly therapeutic raw food diet. Embrace it, and let the healing begin.

—Brenda Davis, RD
co-author of The Kick Diabetes Cookbook, Becoming Raw and Becoming Vegan (Comprehensive and Express Editions)

Dr. Helen Powell-Stoddart provides an excellent blueprint to get your health back on track. Emphasizing the importance of a whole foods plant-based diet, while also providing meal plans and shopping lists to get you started. You have everything you need to revolutionize your health.

—Neal D. Barnard, MD, FACC
Adjunct Associate Professor of Medicine, George Washington University School of Medicine
President, Physicians Committee

It is time to take charge of your health

Take charge of type 2 Diabetes

The goal of **Reverse it!** is to...

- Provide a supported detoxification plan to jumpstart your goal of reversing type 2 diabetes on the fast track
- Provide a 40-day plan to reverse type 2 diabetes
- Provide information about the proper food choices to increase insulin sensitivity
- Provide the benefits of detoxification to reverse type 2 diabetes
- Provide the proper nutrients to support both phase 1 and phase 2 of the liver detoxification process

Reverse it!

For so long, it has been the prevailing thought that type 2 diabetes is a long-term, irreversible chronic disease that can only be "controlled" or "managed" and not reversed. Numerous studies have now scientifically proven that type 2 diabetes can be reversed using a lifestyle plan that includes the proper disease reversing foods, the proper insulin sensitivity improving exercises and the proper balance. **Reverse it!** focuses on a detoxification plan to jumpstart this process by providing the proper nutrition for the cells to recover and perform the way they were intended to. Our goal is to reduce or eliminate the need for chronic medications and reduce the risk of long-term complications of type 2 diabetes and other chronic diseases.

Coming Soon!

Reset

The Genesis Plan- What To Do Next

Forty, The 40-Day Detox Devotional

Forty, The 40-Day Detox Devotional Companion Journal

Dr. Helen is available for speaking engagements on this and other topics. Contact events@p2whealth.com.

Pain 2 Wellness Healthcare
www.pain2wellnesshealthcare.com
www.p2whealth.com

This book is dedicated to my "favorite husband", John Stoddart, without whom I would not have completed this project. His music soothes me and sends me clarity and he makes all my work beautiful. Thank you so very much. To my children for having faith in me and for my incredible patients who sought me out and stayed with me during my transition. You are all appreciated.

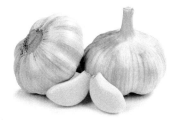

Table of Contents

Preface

Reverse it! is designed to be a 40-day program. This program includes foods that encourage a healthy detoxification process to jumpstart your reversal of type 2 diabetes and other chronic diseases. It is through detoxification that the body will rid itself of unwanted toxins that accumulate in the body and various organs (including the pancreas and liver) that impair the normal processes of metabolism. During this time, the cells of the body will have an opportunity to recover and will start to function correctly. Drinking plenty of water is extremely important in this process.

The first part of the detoxification begins with juicing for 10 days followed by 30 days of raw foods. I encourage you to use as many organic, nonGMO foods as possible to ensure that you consume only natural food that is not tainted or that is minimally tainted by chemicals. Raw plant-based foods are exceptional for the detoxification process providing the necessary nutrition to support both phase 1 and phase 2 of detoxification. Food enzymes are released when food is chewed or otherwise ground up. These food enzymes may help to breakdown foods before we actually begin eating, in the mouth and in the upper part of the stomach (1).

Juicing allows for a faster, more efficient way to absorb life-enhancing, essential nutrients to bathe the cells of the body for increased nourishment. When you juice, the natural fiber found in these foods is purposefully removed to allow for increased absorption of vital nutrients for optimal health. The digestive enzymes in raw foods that are found in our juicing and raw food program allow for better absorption of immune accelerating nutrients found naturally in fruits and vegetables.

The recipes have been designed to support the first phase of liver detoxification that involves the cytochrome P450 system. Phase 1 produces some pretty serious intermediate metabolites that can be even more dangerous than the original toxins.

Our recipes are designed to provide essential antioxidants to neutralize the intermediate metabolites from phase 1 detoxification. This will, subsequently, supply neutralized metabolites to phase 2 detoxification allowing water-soluble products to be excreted from the body through urine and feces. Consuming plenty of clean water is essential.

The program allows for flexibility. There are many recipes to choose from, so there is no set food for breakfast, lunch or dinner. Instead, the menus are interchangeable to prevent boredom (my sister is easily bored, lol). You can be confident to choose any juice for the first 10 days. After juicing, and the following weeks of the detox plan, you can select any food from any of the subsequent categories as well as the juicing program. Please note that some foods have progressively more texture to promote interest. It is best to start with the simple foods and preserve the foods with more texture to later in the detoxification process.

It takes 14 days to change your palate, so the foods chosen take this into consideration. It also takes 21 days to "begin" to form a habit when it comes to food choices. Our goal is to improve your palate from the greasy, fried, salty, and overly sweetened foods of the Standard American Diet (SAD) to a more nutritious, satisfying palate. You will be surprised how your usual level of saltiness or sweetness is reset based on this palate change. It is quite amazing. Foods that were of "normal SAD saltiness" now become too salty and foods of "normal SAD sweetness" become too sweet. I experienced this first hand with my first detoxification in 1995. After 21 days, some of the habits learned during this process will be prohibitive from going back to the typical SAD.

Also, we have included sample meal plans and shopping lists for your convenience. We have even provided a template to build your own shopping lists. These are only samples so, please do not become overwhelmed with the details. The goal is to choose foods that interest you. The savory juices are my personal favorites. Aim to eliminate or decrease unnecessary sugars. Each week, increase the food textures you partake from. It is a gradual increase in food complexity.

You may experience detoxification symptoms such as headaches, nausea, fatigue, flu-like symptoms, gas and bloating. After these symptoms dissipate, you will have more energy, stamina, and better sleep. At the end of the 40 days, your body will be transformed. You will feel incredible and look amazing.

We have provided the recipes in this simple book to accomplish your goals. We focus on detoxifying the liver to allow the body to reset itself in preparation to overcome the "challenge" of type 2 diabetes. All of the recipes have been carefully designed to support both Phase 1 and Phase 2 detoxification in the liver (see chapter 7). Once detoxification occurs and the cells of the body have an opportunity to recover, the principles of this lifestyle transformation will ensue providing a prohibitive platform for type 2 diabetes to ever raise its ugly head again.

As with this and any other program that you begin, please include your doctor so that your blood sugar levels, blood pressure, weight and cholesterol levels are monitored so that medications can be changed, adjusted or eliminated as needed. Your doctor only wants the best for you, so he/she will be happy to see that you are making a change and commanding charge of your health.   Your doctor will be pleased.

Here are a few tips to remember during your detoxification process:

1. Look for products that are a part of the nonGMO verified food project and preferably organic (see figure i). Organic foods can be found in traditional grocery venues as well as specialty organic stores (which tend to be more expensive). Consider becoming a part of a co-op or farmer's market for organic foods. Here you will find more economical pricing. Traditional grocery stores are carrying more organic products. Shop around.

2. During the juicing portion, it is vital to drink your juice every 2-2.5 hours to satisfy hunger pangs. This will amount to about six (6) 16 oz juices daily.

3. Make a list of the week's food plan that you have chosen and shop accordingly.

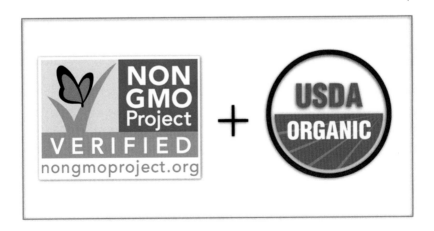

Figure i

4.   Drink fresh, clean water between juices and throughout the day.

5.   You will urinate a lot releasing toxins in the process.

6.   Get plenty of rest aiming to get into bed by 9 pm, if possible.

7.   Aim to walk 30-60 minutes daily, especially for the first 10 days, then progress to a supervised light exercise routine.

8. Ensure your doctor knows that you are changing your lifestyle so that he/she can support you through it and monitor your fasting blood sugar levels, HbA1c, cholesterol, and blood pressure.   You will need your doctor to make some adjustments to all or most of your medications, particularly if you are on insulin or blood pressure medications.

9. Eliminate processed foods, added oils, caffeine, and animal products.

10.Use body products without parabens, phthalates or pore-clogging elements. Try Our Body Detox Line that includes Detox Shower Gel, Detox Body Lotion, Detox Body Scrub, and Detox Body Deodorant.

Type 2 diabetes is reversible if approached correctly. Detoxification is a fabulous way to jumpstart your success. I have seen it happen again and again. Now it's your turn. **Reverse it!**

Introduction

I was in medical school when I lost my mother. It was the hardest thing I have ever had to deal with. Before my mom became sick, the worse thing I had to deal with was how many times my ex-boyfriend would be unfaithful to me. He was like a broken record.

"I am so sorry, it was a mistake. It will never happen again..."

Don't judge. I was young and foolish. Still, I would suffer that heartbreak a thousand times out of a thousand if it meant I could have my mother back. Dealing with an unfaithful boyfriend was nothing compared to the pain I felt when I lost my precious jewel.

She was diagnosed with Diabetes in the 1980s. Back then people called it "a little sugar." I was young, but somehow I knew that despite the cute name, it would mean big trouble later. I was right. I would carefully monitor my mother's eating while we were together and she would comply. Eventually, however, my voice was drowned by my dad and 6 older siblings who would invariably say, "Oh, let her have it. It's just a little ..."

They didn't understand the connection between diet and health and truthfully, I didn't either at the time. I just knew something was wrong with having a poor diet and "a little sugar."

That "it's just a little ..." ended up causing my mom to need several medications to control her diabetes, hypertension and high cholesterol. Then came Lasix to treat the developing heart failure. It wasn't long before the self-administered medications ceased to be effective. Her heart could no longer handle even minimal activity. Intermittent hospital stays became more long-term necessities to have the fluid around her heart professionally removed to improve and control her breathing.

I would call my mom every day from DC to talk to her and to make sure she was ok. We all did. She always had good advice for me, and was such an incredible inspiration.

I had another reason for checking in on her, though. I was now a medical student at The Howard University School of Medicine and was learning more and more about the heart every day.

I remember speaking to my Cardiology Attending Physician about my mother's condition. I still remember the tears that helplessly escaped my eyes when he said the words that no loving daughter ever wants to hear. "Your mother is going to die." Those words still ring in my ears piercing my heart each time I recall them.

He was right. My mother's hospitalizations became more frequent. As a matter of fact, she spent more time in the hospital than she spent at home during that last year. I was nervous and preoccupied with what was going on at home with my mother. It made it difficult at times to concentrate on the lectures about the anatomical heart when my own emotional heart was in such turmoil.

I thought to take a leave from medical school for a while, but she wouldn't have it. So, from school

672 miles away, I continued to worry while I studied about her heart condition.

Then, one cold day in November, the phone rang. "Mom is in the hospital," my sister whispered from behind an avalanche of tears. "She coded, and they have rushed her to the hospital." She was there, in the hospital, with my daddy and 5 of my older siblings. I, along with my two other sisters, who also lived in DC, soberly got into my sister's car and drove to Indiana on one of the most dangerous days of the season. The drive was long, arduous and even dangerous at times. It was scary, but we were determined to get there as quickly as possible to see her and touch her.

I was afraid—very afraid. I saw my Cardiology Attending's words replaying in my mind's eye. I was anxious. We all were. I was worried that I would miss seeing her alive. I am sure my sisters thought the same, but we didn't speak of it. We kept our conversations positive and faithful.

However, I was secretly concerned that she would be hooked up to tubes and machines and we would have to make an unthinkable decision. I would never be able to do that. All kinds of horrible thoughts flooded my mind—some real and others imagined, but all were devastating as we drove through the first blizzard of the season from Washington, DC to our home in Indiana.

We arrived at the hospital late that evening and entered her hospital room. At first, she was unable to communicate with us, but then she improved. Later, when she was able to speak, she told us about the dream she had when she was unconscious.

She described a white light and spoke of speaking to God. She asked Him if she could see His face. He told her no because it was not her time. She really wanted to see His face. He warned her, "your children are not ready, and no one has ever seen my face and lived to tell about it. You must go back". And she did.

She came back to us. She said that at the end of her dream, God showed her each of her children coming into her hospital room in a particular order. When she opened her eyes, she saw that we had indeed entered in the exact order that she had dreamt.

Now she was awake, but very afraid. I didn't pick up on that then, but many years later, after seeing it happen to other near-death hospitalized patients, I can look back and tell that she didn't want to go to sleep even though she was exhausted. She was afraid that if she closed her eyes, she wouldn't open them again.

Talk about a lot of praying. I don't think I had ever prayed as much as I did during that time both on the road and in the hospital room. We really were not ready for any of it. We definitely needed more time with her. I really needed her.

I needed to talk to her and ask her questions that had not yet arisen in my mind about life. I needed to hear her voice calling my name and telling me she loved me as many times as I could. I wanted to smell her hands that often smelled of onions and garlic as she prepped dinner. I wanted to see and feel her touch. I wanted to remember what she felt like. I needed her to know that I still needed her. She needed to know how much I loved her and treasured her. I just needed her. You may not understand my feelings if you still have your mother, but there are others of you out there that can feel my pain. The needs that I had all take time and 27 years was just not enough.

Even now, I have a cassette tape (don't laugh) from the answering machine I had then that has her voice recorded on it. I started saving all of her voice messages. I treasure that cassette. It is locked up in a briefcase that she gave me for medical school. I keep it stored away, but close enough to open when I need to remember her voice—when I need a "fix."

Praise God she survived. For a time, at least. I think God was preparing us for what was to come in our near future. Her husband and 8 children weren't ready that day.

We stayed at home through her recovery and her release from the hospital with only a slight understanding of her frailty. I remember taking tons of pictures with her. We took turns kissing her, hugging her, sitting close and holding her. It was all captured on film so we would remember her and she would know how much we loved her.

When it was time to go, we were so afraid to leave because, in our hearts, we knew it would be the last time we would see her alive.

Six months later on July 24, 1993, I got an envelope from the American Board of Examiners. My scores for Part 1 of my medical boards were inside.   I was very nervous because I couldn't remember if a "pass" notification would be a large envelope or a small one. The thought of it made me afraid to open the jacket because I wasn't quite sure if I had passed the exam or not.

Part I of the boards is the most difficult one of all the ones I would have to take in the future and I was nervous—exceptionally nervous.   I needed "my mommy".

I waited until Saturday night. I called my mom from my apartment in DC so she could talk me through it. With her close by (at least by phone), I was able to open the envelope and, to my excitement, I passed!   I was screaming and jumping up and down when I heard her say, "I knew you would pass. I had no doubt. I know you will do anything you put your mind to. I am so proud of you." She was always so proud of me and always so encouraging. She was my biggest fan and my best cheerleader.

In celebration of my boards, I went to LA on the following Monday to "hang out" with my friend Lilyan. I didn't want my mom to know that I was traveling because she only worry until I returned in a couple of days. I didn't want to upset her.

Lilyan and I had a great time at Redondo Beach enjoying the sunshine as we devoured our favorite ice cream flavors and inhaled the view of the water and the people milling about. We did a little shopping as we walked.

Later that evening, we went back to her house. After about an hour or so, the phone rang. It was my sister and my "boyfriend" on the line. He's the one I told you about before. I heard his voice say, "she's gone. Mom died, Helen. She's gone. She was rushed to the hospital, but it was already too late."

I screamed and cried so loud that Lilyan's mother ran to me and held me. I was in total disbelief. She had been doing so well. Even though she coded the November before this, I was somehow under the impression that if I didn't see her sickness, it wouldn't exist. The human psyche is very interesting.

Lilyan's mother mothered me that night and even let me lay next to her as I cried myself to sleep. It was like a bad dream, but I wasn't waking up from it.

Lilyan made all the arrangements to get me back home and even had one of our doctor friends prescribe 2 Valium for me to handle what was going to happen over the next few days. I still remember the tears that I had become all too familiar with. Even now my eyes well up when I remember that moment— that night I got the call.

She was buried on August 2, 1993. It was my nephew's birthday. What a horrible memory for him. He loved his grandmother. He was 14 years old. I almost felt worse for him than myself.

On a side note, five years later, I got married to my "favorite husband" on August 2, 1998. That way, my nephew would have a better memory on his birthday—his aunt's wedding instead of his grandmother's funeral.

Shortly after my mom's death, we found out that my father had developed prostate cancer—again. He had been diagnosed when I was in high school. He had a surgical procedure back then to remove the malignancy. They had gotten it all, but it came back. It came back with a vengeance. It had metastasized to his colon, liver, lungs and bone. Actually, we were not sure of the primary site of the cancer at the time—I don't think we ever did. We didn't know if it was prostate or colon, but we knew it was everywhere. We were devastated and desperate. We had just lost our mother and we were certainly not ready to lose him too.

He decided to undergo treatment at the famed Mayo Clinic in Minnesota. My sister Jackie, went with him. His chest X-ray revealed that the disease had taken a major foothold in his lungs. I still remember my sister's words to me that day. She said, "my daddy is going to die." We all called him "my daddy." It has confused many. One of my friends asked if we all had the same dad because we all said he was *my* daddy.   For the record, we did.

At any rate, *my* daddy began chemotherapy and hated it.   The treatments turned his nails black and kept him feeling sick.   We hated to see him suffer so much, but we knew it was a necessary treatment.

In an effort to make him more comfortable and to handle the treatments, we did some research and found a place in California that espoused a whole-food, plant-based lifestyle using raw foods, juicing and wheatgrass.   We hoped the increased nutrition would help him tolerate the chemo better because it was taking a toll on him.

He had become extremely weak when my sister, Leacadia, took him to the place in California and checked him in.   We chose an in-house program that would last a total of 3 weeks. I spoke to him on the phone when he arrived. He sounded downcast and disheartened and I imagine he felt a lot like he sounded. I am not sure what any of us expected the outcome would be, but we needed to do something.

The program was very comprehensive and included a *complete* lifestyle change. It was totally different from his previous meat and potatoes life. He walked daily in the early morning fresh air, exercised, slept and relaxed. He ate only raw plants, and juiced his own wheatgrass. There were classes and seminars on this new lifestyle he was learning to adapt to. It was a *huge* change for him.

After two weeks, I called him again and the difference in his voice was remarkable. He sounded energetic and optimistic. "Dad, how are you?", I said.

"I feel great!"

"What do you mean? What happened?"

"I got a lot of exercise and they fed me food I have never seen before." I laughed in relief. I was elated.

My dad left that facility and continued the new lifestyle that he embraced for the upcoming weeks. He was doing well. His doctors were amazed. They had given him months to live and not only was he surviving, he was thriving.

I remember they asked him what he was doing. He told them about the program. They were very supportive and said, "whatever you are doing, just keep doing it." He was able to tolerate the shot that he received for chemo much better with this improved lifestyle.

Three years later, my father remarried. His new wife started cooking for him and he slowly began reverting to his old diet of meat and potatoes. We repeatedly informed her (and reminded him) that this was the very lifestyle that brought on the cancer that had almost taken his life (2).

They didn't seem to comprehend. Even plans to go back to the facility in California for a "refresher" failed, repeatedly. I believe my father felt that he was healed and that perhaps his diet didn't have as much to do with his recovery as he had thought. Maybe he was just depressed. I know he missed my mom.

On December 24, 2003, I had my second child. She was my Christmas present. All of my immediate family, including my dad, came to Maryland in anticipation of her birth. She was actually supposed to be born on December 21, but she waited until Christmas Eve.

It was wonderful for my family to be there. My dad got a chance to hold her and kiss on her. He loved babies. She was "chunky" so she was a lot to love. He had a great time with both of my girls.

I am so incredibly happy that he had an opportunity to meet my baby and spend time with my oldest child though they remember very little to nothing about him. My oldest daughter was just over 2 years old when he lost the battle in April of 2004 and my baby was just 4 months old. Returning to the "Standard American Diet" I believe, cost him in the end. I still remember where I was when I got the news of the second call I never wanted to receive.

My husband was buying a few items from BJ's Food Warehouse in Bowie, MD. I was in the parking lot nursing my baby in the car while my 2 1/2 year-old slept.

I felt helpless again. I had just lost my other parent. I was not a child, but I felt orphaned. We all felt orphaned, even though we were all grown by this time.

Even with all I had learned during my incredible medical school education at Howard University and the fabulous training I received in my combined residency of Internal Medicine and Physical Medicine and Rehabilitation, at The Johns Hopkins/Sinai Hospital Program, I couldn't save him.   At that moment, drowning in grief, I felt sorry for myself and my siblings. It was the second hardest thing in my life.   Medical School and 2 residency training programs were a breeze in comparison. Delivering babies was nothing.

Nonetheless, he had defied metastatic disease for 11 years. Eleven years was much more than the months he had been given.

Even though he had lived longer than any of us had imagined, it still made it difficult to hear the words— "my daddy just died." I was devastated and I cried like a baby right there in the parking lot. Some things you just never forget.

He had been doing quite well until he reverted to the old way of eating. I have since learned that it is very likely that the Standard American Diet (SAD) of meat and dairy that crept back into his life is likely the culprit of his death (2, 3).

Time will never heal the loss of my parents, but it has given me perspective and purpose. I got to see first-hand, especially in my dad's life, how powerful a plant-based diet really is. I started adopting that lifestyle and committed myself to learning as much as I could. I told several of my friends who had cancer about my dad's experience and those who changed to a plant-based lifestyle with their treatment lived and those who continued their animal-based lifestyle died shortly after their diagnosis. The plant-based food connection was solidified in my mind through these experiences.

Did you know that a plant-based diet is powerful enough to reverse type 2 diabetes, hypertension, hypercholesterolemia, lupus, cardiovascular disease and so many other diet exacerbated illness whether it runs in your family or not?

My mother had type 2 diabetes, congestive heart failure, hypercholesterolemia, obesity and hypertension. My dad had cancer, hypertension and diabetes. Scary.

In addition, two of my sisters have diabetes, 5 have hypertension or have had blood pressure issues—also scary. My only brother died due to heart failure and all of its complications, but his was due to his lifestyle habits that I begged him to change. The people around you really suffer the most. It is so difficult to lose a sibling and another family member. He was the third of my closest relatives to die. We miss him so much. We miss all of them. It is difficult to express in words.

I definitely needed the changes I made in my own lifestyle. I started the plant-based lifestyle journey in 1995 and though it was very difficult in the early days, I have never regretted it. A healthier lifestyle has paid off for me and saved money for us.

Apparently, insurance companies use your family history (essentially your genes) sometimes to determine your insurance premium.

My husband and I applied for Whole Life Insurance. We had Term Life Insurance, but wanted to convert it while we were still young. Our broker gave us several options for insurance companies to chose from. We decided to go with company B. We had viewed their benefits and pricing and it looked attractive.

A representative came to our house and had us complete the paperwork and did all of the testing according to their policy. As I was completing the paperwork, I noticed that one of the questions was "have you had a close family member to die prior to the age of 60 due to heart disease?" I sighed sadly as I marked the answer yes. I had to explain that it was my mother who had passed at age 59.

A few days later, we received a letter in the mail accepting us as new policy owners. When we looked at the premium, we noticed that my premium was 3 times the amount previously quoted. I didn't understand why, so I asked.

They reported that my policy premium was higher because of my family history—my genes. It didn't matter to them that I didn't have any of the conditions my mom had. They didn't ask about my lifestyle to know that it was completely different from my parents. They didn't make the correlation that by the time my mother was my age, she had already been diagnosed with diabetes and hypertension.

All of my tests were normal. My blood pressure was normal and had never been elevated. I had had 2 babies and never had gestational diabetes. All of my labs that were drawn were normal. Why would my premium be so high? My family history had anything to do with me, but they believed otherwise.

I penned a letter to the company explaining my position while explaining why I was declining their insurance. "I will just have to stay with the term policy that I already have," I wrote. Since we had the policy for such a long time, the premium was a lot less and I wasn't willing to pay so much more unfairly.

They reviewed the policy and my data and, after some deliberation, they reversed their decision decreasing my premium to its original estimate.

I have certainly been dealt with the "raw end of the gene pool," but while having the "gene" for diabetes, obesity, hypertension or any other chronic disease does increase the risk for these conditions to develop (as the insurance companies obviously know), it's the lifestyle that more often determines if you actually get the disease ("challenge") or not. In other words, your genes load the "gun", but your lifestyle pulls the "trigger."

T.Colin Campbell of the China Study, as well as others who have studied this subject, have now determined that disease causing genes can be turned off (3). We have discovered a way of living and eating that promotes health, defies age, enhances and boosts moods and creates energy!

Energy is very important. I seem to have lots of it. I have been known to go to work all day in a busy medical practice, drive home, cook dinner, put the kids to bed and paint parts of my house while the rest of my family slept. I actually faux painted my home office, two bathrooms, our bedroom, sitting room and our piano room all by myself and all after full workdays.

I certainly don't recommend that, but it brings me great peace to paint my house and step back and say "I did that." It is one of the things that brings me satisfaction and pleasure. You have to treat yourself to things that bring you satisfaction, pleasure and peace. Ok, so painting doesn't bring you peace. I get it.

What brings you peace, satisfaction and pleasure? Whatever constructive activity brings you joy and peace, have at it! I hope that doesn't include eating the Standard American Diet. Just sayin'.

My sister teases me about all that I do after work all the time. She says "who does all that after work?"

She came to me one day in the most sincere tone and asked, "Can doctors write narcotic pill prescriptions for themselves?"

"No," I replied. "We could lose our license for writing those kind of medications for ourselves."

"Then what about their friends? Can their friends write prescriptions for them?"

"No, then they could lose their license too."

Then she asked me a question I will never forget. "Where do you get your drugs from?"

"What?"

"You must be on something because you have too much energy!"

We both laughed hysterically. She was right about one thing—I do have tons of energy. It comes from my diet.

Since then, my sister has added more plant foods to her diet and she reports better sleep, weight loss, increased energy, healthier hair and a general feeling of well-being. I can tell you that she is less stressed and that is always a good thing.

Well, I've shared with you a bit of my own personal journey and you may be thinking to yourself, "that's good for her, but it will never work for me." I encourage you to give it a try.

No one has the corner on the market for well-being. You can have it too!

The **Reverse it!** program is your guide along the path to increased health and wellness. I have developed this plan to jumpstart you on the road to reverse type 2 diabetes. By following the plan that I have created, backed by years of research and personal experience, you will have more energy, better health, incredible sleep and an amazing feeling of well-being—and that is always a great thing. Start now! **Reverse it!**

The Background

Chapter 1

An Epidemic

According to the Centers for Disease Control and Prevention (CDC), diabetes is prevalent. In the US, 29.1 million people have diabetes and 8.1 million people are undiagnosed. That means that over 9.3% of people in our country have diabetes right now. As a matter of fact, over 25.9% of people over the age of 65 are plagued with this dreaded condition (4). Unfortunately, the numbers continue to grow in our country and abroad.

Of all the cases of diabetes, 90% have type 2 diabetes. It is the seventh leading cause of death in the world according to the World Health Organization's 2016 statistics. It was not even on the global list in 2000 (5).

When my mother was diagnosed with diabetes, they called it a "little sugar." Diabetes is not the benign, "just a little sugar" problem. Instead, it comes with a myriad of complications that I have experienced first hand.

Diabetes is the leading cause of kidney failure, non-traumatic lower limb amputations, the leading cause of new cases of blindness among adults in the US, and a significant cause of heart disease and stroke (5).

As you can see, the complications can be deadly and affect many systems including the kidneys, legs, eyes, heart, brain, and even nerves. It is interesting that the underlying culprit of uncontrolled blood sugars can be reversed eliminating the risk of these vicious, long-term complications.

Controlling blood glucose levels is of the utmost importance because, over time, high blood glucose levels can damage both small and large blood vessels in the body. When uncontrolled glucose damages small vesicles we call it microvascular complications and when they damage large vessels we call them macrovascular complications (6).

The microvascular complications are why diabetics are prone to cataracts and glaucoma, which can both lead to blindness. Damage to the blood vessels of the kidneys leads to kidney failure and when it affects the nerves, it leads to peripheral neuropathy.

The macrovascular complications may lead to a heart attack, stroke or damage to the blood vessels of the legs causing a condition called peripheral vascular disease. Diabetes is not just a "little sugar." It is a costly disease to your health and your pocket.

The financial burden of diabetes and its complications are forever increasing. People with diabetes spend greater than 2 times more money for their healthcare obligations than people without diabetes. The national cost of diabetes in the United States in 2012 was more than $245 billion, which is 71 billion more dollars than just 5 years before. The financial burden and the individual and family burden is likely part of the reason why the American Diabetes Association's Mission is to prevent and cure diabetes and to improve the lives of all people affected by diabetes (7).

Indeed, the burden on families and finances is overwhelming, but the financial burden is not where my concern is. My concern is more about the tremendous and immeasurable toll that it takes on families and loved ones. Mine included.

Chapter 2

It's in the Genes

I lost my mother to complications of diabetes. She had hypertension, high cholesterol, and heart disease. She died with heart failure, but the MI (heart attack) is what took her life at only age 59.

When my mom passed, I had not yet met my husband, married or had children. At our wedding, my 3 older sisters read a tribute to my mother as her representatives since I wasn't fortunate enough to have her there. When I was in the hospital having my first child, my sister Anita, thoughtfully enlarged a picture of my mother and hung it in my hospital room. That was as close as I could get to her. It really helped.

My father had metastatic prostate or colon cancer and died of a PE (blood clot in his lungs). He also had diabetes. He was only 75.

My mother's massive family of 12 lost most of their family members to diabetes, heart disease or a combination or complications of both. One of my favorite aunts had the difficulty of peripheral neuropathy. She had minimal sensation especially in her feet and legs due to her diabetes. She was also morbidly obese. One day she got in the bathtub and didn't realize that the water was extremely hot, and it caused her skin to burn. She died of complications from the burns.

My mother's youngest living sister had type 2 diabetes along with high cholesterol and hypertension. She lost one of her legs to a non-healing diabetic ulcer. She was in the 85% of people with diabetes who have major amputations. I was concerned that she would lose her other leg since 50% of diabetics will have a second amputation on the opposite limb. Instead, the heart disease claimed her life first.

One study showed that following an amputation, up to 50% of people with diabetes will die within 2 years (8). "Yep." That was my aunt. Another aunt died from breast cancer years before. I have one aunt left, and she has diabetes. They all had similar diets.

Among my own siblings, 2 have diabetes (I wrote my program for them), and a few of my other sisters either have had or are dealing with high blood pressure.

My brother was different. He was a recovering alcoholic and died of alcoholic cardiomyopathy. He was only 58.

I miss him so much. Losing a sibling is odd. It's even weirder to have lost now 3 close family members. I can hardly believe it. It 's like a nightmare that I can't wake up from.

We all had the same diet growing up of course. There were no special meals made if you didn't like something. My father's favorite line was "you will eat it before it eats you." That is the same rule I use in my family.

My parents had similar diets to their siblings growing up but, even though they changed their diet to a no-pork and no-shelled fish diet, they still developed diet-exacerbated illnesses. Why? I was confused.

When my father developed metastatic cancer in 1993, we were devastated. It was the same year we lost my mother. His cancer metastasized to his lungs and liver, and the primary cause was thought to be either his prostate or colon. We were never sure.

My dad started chemo at the amazing Mayo Clinic in Minnesota, but had difficulty tolerating it. To help him, we decided to do some research, and we found a plant-based program in California for people like him with cancer and other illnesses. Even though I was a vegetarian, it was the first time I learned about a plant-based diet and the process of detoxification. I was amazed at the results.

My dad went there for 3 weeks, and when he left there and went back to the Mayo Clinic for follow up, the doctors were very pleased with his results and encouraged him to keep doing what he was doing.

My dad lived an additional 11 years on a plant-based diet. Unfortunately, in his last year, he returned to his old way of living—a diet of meat, fish, and potatoes. He died not long after that.

The power of plant-based foods is incredible. My dad did well as long as he consumed mostly plants. He became sick when he returned to the Standard American Diet (SAD).

After seeing how well he was doing on this new lifestyle of plant-based foods, I decided to try it for myself. I went to the same facility a couple of years after he did and participated in my first detoxification program. That was in 1995.

Many years later, I started piecing together the puzzle that had confused me so many years before. I thought about my dad and how successfully he thrived after his diagnosis on a detoxification program and plant-based diet. I thought about the fact that I was never plagued with diabetes, heart disease, obesity or breast cancer like my family genes dictated. I was struck by the fact that I was the only one in my family that changed my diet and the only one to have participated in a detox other than my dad. Could detoxification have anything to do with it? I mean, I have the same genes they do.

I know about having bad genes. I have them. I am very sensitive to the people who say "it runs in my family." However, I now know that your genes give you a propensity—sort of a suggestion, —loads the gun, but your lifestyle pulls the trigger. Your lifestyle can cause you to develop the disease. In plain words, you can treat a pair of Versace jeans poorly and lose them, and manage a pair of Target jeans with care and preserve them. Your health works the same way. Treat your body well and your body will treat you well. You only get one body after all, and only one set of your given genes. Why beat them up?

Chapter 3

What's Fat Got To Do With It?

Let's look at the function of insulin and investigate what it has to do with type 2 diabetes. To do this, we need to start with the basics.

The basic unit of life is called the cell. It is the building block of life. Anything that is living is made up of cells. Some organisms are made of one cell, while others are made of many. The human body, for instance, is made up of trillions of cells—approximately 37.2 trillion. That's a lot of cells!

The outside of the cell is surrounded by something called a cell or plasma membrane that is like a skin to protect the cell.

The cell membrane separates the outside environment of the cell from the inside environment of the cell. It ensures that the two environments maintain their differences.

Cells also have "organelles" or little organs inside each of them. The function of the organelles is to assist in the "busyness" of the cell based on how the cell is programmed and what functions it will have. It performs activities that support life, from the building of proteins, to duplicating itself through mitosis, to energy production.

Randomly distributed along the cell membrane are openings called channels. The channels are communication sites from the inside of the cell to the outside of the cell, and house proteins called transmembrane proteins. The channels are for the entry and exit of substances into and out of the cell. This system allows much needed nutrients to enter the cell, while encouraging unneeded materials or waste to exit the cell. One such substance that is needed by the cell is glucose.

One of the purposes of the channels is to house the transport protein called Glut-4 that is to be transported to the surface of the cell, where it provides a place or entrance for glucose. Glucose is the preferred source of ATP or energy production.

When glucose metabolism is working properly, glucose comes into the cell from the bloodstream escorted by insulin, which is produced in pancreatic beta cells. The glucose is then broken down by mitochondria—the "power plant" of the cell, to produce energy.

In type 2 diabetes, where glucose metabolism is not working properly, glucose is unable to enter the cell from the bloodstream. The cell becomes resistant to insulin and refuses its request for glucose entry. Without the help of insulin, the cells are unable to utilize glucose and to produce enough energy for survival. Glucose then accumulates in the bloodstream.

This phenomenon is called insulin resistance. Insulin resistance is one of the hallmarks of type 2 diabetes. Insulin is not able to escort the glucose into the cell to perform its tasks.

When glucose is unable to be taken into the cells, too much of it starts to accumulate in the bloodstream. This can lead to serious damage to the blood vessels of the body leading to blindness, kidney failure, and heart disease.

Imagine you are glucose and you are going to an event where everyone is invited, but there is only limited space. You are the life of the party. You are the one that brings the energy to the room. However, your entrance is inhibited by something blocking the door that keeps it closed.

The door is closed because, now, there is standing room only, and the fire department has banned further attendees from entering the space. There is no room left for even one more attendee no matter who you are.

In this instance, you—glucose, the preferred guest, are left outside of the room with no way to enter. Your escort thinks that if he can get more of his friends to help, he can get you inside the door, but the door is jammed. The party is, resistant to your escort and therefore, resistant to you. You are now angry because you got all dressed up with nowhere to go that you go out with rage and cause damage to other parties. That's the non-scientific explanation.

Scientific evidence reveals that increased levels of plasma lipids, especially free fatty acids (FFA) and triglycerides, are important in insulin resistance (25, 26). This idea was first introduced in the

1960's when Randle and his group (26) showed that there was a competition with FFA and plasma glucose to be used as fuel for energy production.

These FFA are essentially filling up the space inside the cell so that glucose can not enter the cell, even though insulin is asking nicely.

Since glucose cannot enter the cell, energy levels are lowered, fatigue ensues, insulin levels and blood glucose levels increase.

Neal Barnard describes this process as a "gummed-up lock". This shows that the ability of insulin to escort glucose into the cell, is blocked by the accumulation of something within the cells. Studies have shown that this something is fat (18).

Studies also show that it doesn't take a long time for the fat to accumulate in the cell. It is noted that this accumulation begins in muscle in as little as 3 days according to Pennington Biomedical Research Center (27).

This is called intramyocellular lipids. It has been shown, in this study, that the genes that produce mitochondria (the power house —fat burners) were turned off by fatty foods. The mitochondria are inhibited from burning fat with fat as the cell becomes overwhelmed with fat accumulation (27).

Intramyocellular lipids or intramyocellular fat is what prevents glucose from entering the cell even when escorted by insulin. It is what "gums-up the lock".

The result of intramyocellular lipids or fat is an accumulation of glucose in the bloodstream that then damages the blood vessels and leads to blindness, kidney failure and even heart disease.

Chapter 4

Anti-Aging?

In 1995, as a senior medical student, I had my first encounter with plant-based foods as a lifestyle habit. No, the sexy term, "plant-based" wasn't in vogue yet, but plants, indeed, were.

As I mentioned several times before, my father was diagnosed with metastatic cancer with the primary being either his colon or prostate and was given months to live. He was on chemotherapy and was followed at the esteemed Mayo Clinic in Rochester, Minnesota. He was not tolerating the chemo very well and was very sick and very fatigued.

You must understand that my dad was a straight "meat and potatoes" kind of guy, but he always knew he needed to do better.

When we were growing up, he would declare at least once a month that we were going to stop eating meat and eat more vegetables—become vegetarian.

"As soon as all this meat is out of the freezer, we are going to be vegetarian," he would say.

I remember my mom following his directive at least twice. She would use up all the meat in the freezer and fill up on vegetables (canned back then, lol). She would fix his breakfast, lunch or dinner without meat and all vegetables. He would take one look at the plate and say, "where's my meat?" Yep, a real meat and potatoes man. The next grocery store trip ended up with a basket heavy on the meat again.

The only fresh vegetables I recall eating on a regular basis while growing up were greens and string beans. Salads were 1-2 times a week, but not a regular part of our meals. At any rate, my dad was used to the Standard American Diet (SAD). He didn't want to change, but we knew he needed to. We didn't know how to go about making the change but knew he had to.

In our desperation for him to tolerate his chemo better, we researched and researched and finally found the facility that encouraged plant-based nutrition. There, he learned all about this approach to health, and it lead my dad to make a complete lifestyle change. The crux of the program involved detoxification, plant-based foods, exercise, and fresh air.

It made such a difference in his life, and the difference started after only 2 weeks. His energy level soared. He sounded and looked like a different person. He looked younger and felt great. The best part was when he returned to the Mayo Clinic for continued treatment, the doctors at the Mayo Clinic were pleasantly surprised. Their words were "whatever you are doing, keep doing it!"

In 1998, 4 years after my father's would-be terminal diagnosis, I married the love of my life and my dad proudly walked me down the aisle. He was very handsome in his black tuxedo and walked upright, in step with me. To look at him, you would not have guessed that he had been given only a few months to live just a few years before. No one would have known what he had been through.

Later, at our reception, one of my girlfriends came up to me and said, "ooh girl, your daddy is fine!"

I said, "leave my daddy alone. He is 70 years old!" Lol!

He looked very young. I had already noticed that particular feature about him. I thought to myself, I wonder if the food has anything to do with it? My dad was the oldest of 5 children, and he literally looked like the youngest.

In 1995, I had an opportunity to go to the same place and experience the same program that my dad participated in. I did everything they said. It was indeed a challenge for me because I wasn't used to eating this type of food. Though the meals were always beautifully prepared, I didn't know what anything was on my plate. All I knew was that the food was raw and full of vegetables.

At the end of 2 weeks, I felt energized, and my skin was all aglow. We put nothing on our skin that would clog our pores. We did not wear anti-perspirant. Anti-perspiring would prohibit the exit of toxins from the armpits because it is literally an "anti-perspiring" product. Toxins come out in perspiration through the skin. Who knew that these lifestyle changes would have such a profound effect on me. I was already healthy, I thought, but I never had so much energy.

Interestingly, after the 2 weeks of eating this way, they offered a treat. We had the option of having vegetable soup or fruit soup. We all crowded in the dining hall with excitement so that we could be the first to snag a bowl of fruit soup. Most people wanted something sweet (we had nothing sweet for 2 weeks, and nothing had salt in it).

I was one of the ones going for the fruit soup. I hurriedly picked up my soup from the tray and took one sip of it. I couldn't eat it. It seemed like they had put way too much sugar in it and I didn't like it. To our surprise, there was no added sugar. The fruit was merely apples. Apples! The apples were way too sweet for all of us.

It took only 2 weeks of changing my palate that helped me understand that it only takes 2 weeks to break my habit of the SAD. After 2 weeks, the foods that I once consumed voraciously were too sweet or too salty.

I have noticed this with my patients. Usual seasonings become too much. Way too much. This helped me to cut back on the amount of salt and sugar I put on my food. It is really amazing that it happens like that.

Another thing happened to me there too. I used to have the worst menstrual cramps. I had to be picked up from school several times in high school, and I stayed in my room several times in college. I even missed a few events because of my cramps. However, once I detoxed in 1995, I never had cramps again.

I maintained much of the new lifestyle I adopted by at least 90% in the early years. I had already given up red meat, and never ate pork or shelled fish because I knew those were bad for me. But I eventually became entirely plant-based. My energy level remained steady and continues even 23 years later.

I often hear from my patients and my former classmates that I look so young. "You look like one of the kids," some say. I assure you that I don't think I look that young and kids absolutely know that I am my children's mother, but I guess I really don't look my age.

One day, something happened that made me acutely aware of my age though. I started receiving magazines from a company called "Soft Surroundings". I looked at the magazine and admired the "older" women in the catalog. The women looked amazing in their casually clad clothing items. Oh wow! Older, but still so fashionable. I have always considered myself to be fashionable so I could see myself wearing these outfits... when I become an "older" woman. Then about a week later, I received my first solicitation from AARP. AARP? Why are they sending me solicitations?

It hit me like a ton of bricks! Oh! I am turning 50. I *am* an "older" woman! How did they know? Believe me, they know when your birthday is better than you. If you are not yet 50, just wait. It's coming.

But guess what? I don't mind anymore. I carry my AARP card proudly now, and vendors don't usually believe it's mine until I show them my ID. I was also carded by someone that could have been my child when I tried to buy some non-alcoholic sparkling cider! Really?

I discovered that plants actually slow down the aging process by slowing down something we call telomere shortening. Telomere length is a biomarker of aging (9). That happens to be what I have experienced. You can too. I think plants are excellent to eat, but to be anti-aging on top of that? I'm in!

Aside from the anti-aging part, which is an incredible side effect of eating this way, none of the chronic medical conditions that have plagued my family have ever affected me, even during pregnancy. That's a plus!

Chapter 5

A Challenge

One would suspect that gestational diabetes or even hypertension would have shown up in one of my pregnancies, but it never did. Even now, 15 years after my second child was born, my blood pressure has always been in the 1"teens" over about 70, and my blood sugars have always been healthy.

I have certainly been fortunate. I don't say this to brag or to be boastful, but I do know that because my diet is significantly different, I haven't had to deal with chronic illnesses and my family doesn't have to, if they choose, and now, neither do you.

Although my husband has always been supportive, he wasn't on board with the food plan initially. He is now. He doesn't do all that I do, but he enjoys the meals I prepare for him. He is doing better when he travels, and I am so excited about that.

There are so many benefits to choosing a plant-based approach to health. I have learned the importance of diet and its positive or negative effect on health. As a matter of fact, if I knew what I know now before my mother died, I think both my parents would still be alive. They would be on a plant-based diet, and they would still be together living with us. They would have no other choice, but they would enjoy it. Unfortunately, it is not the case, but hey, a girl can dream.

My focus now is to help as many people as I can to avoid the heartache of losing a loved one or loved ones like I have.

The loss of my parents, particularly my mother, hit me extremely hard. I literally had to see a psychologist to help me cope with the loss of her because before then, I had not lost anyone so precious to me.

I still remember walking through the hospital at Howard University Hospital as a 3rd-year medical student, breaking down as my eyes flooded with tears as I walked to my locker outside of the surgical suites. I remember my friend and classmate, Scott, asked, "what's wrong?" "It's my mother," and he said, "I know," empathetically. He hugged me and let me cry on his shoulder that day right there at my locker. I can never forget his kindness.

I cried a lot during my medical school and residency years after she passed. I had just started my clinical studies, so I was going into my third year. It was challenging for me to help other people with their medical issues when I wasn't able to help my own mother. I couldn't bring her back.

I usually tried not to talk to my dad or my siblings when I was having a particularly "weepy" day because I didn't want them to have a "weepy" day if they were ok. So instead, I cried in the Psychologist's office because she was paid to see and hear me cry. I even told her that, and she smiled and just kept handing me tissues. She had such a kind, understanding face.

There was no known cure for diabetes back then, and according to several authorities, there is no cure now, but research is pouring in about the ability to reverse type 2 diabetes and other chronic diseases (10, 11, 12, 13, 14, 15, 16, 17, 18, 19, 20)

I am glad to know that the American Diabetes Association believes that prediabetes is reversible and they report that you can prevent or delay type 2 diabetes by maintaining a healthy weight, eating well and being active (7).

Fortunately, not only is prediabetes reversible, but so is full-blown type 2 diabetes. The same rules apply. Maintain a healthy weight, eat well and be active (1, 10, 11, 12, 19, 20).

Eating well and proper exercise is what I focus on in my practice. A healthy weight just naturally ensues. In my own study and research, I have come across information that has been life-changing for many of my patients. I share this information in the pages that follow in words and in recipes.

We seem to be clear on maintaining a healthy weight and even on the need for exercise, but we often teeter on making the dietary changes that are necessary to reverse type 2 diabetes.

It is interesting to me that the very people who need to make the changes are often the most resistant. They say things like, " I am going to eat my meat or I am not changing my food, I can't go without my meat. How can you eat that stuff", and on and on.

I am not here to convince anyone to become plant-based, but I do know that it has been scientifically proven that a plant-based lifestyle actually reverses many chronic diseases (10, 11, 12, 13, 14, 15, 16, 17, 18, 19, 20). It is a choice. It is your choice.

Most often people don't want to start a plant-based lifestyle because they believe that they have to sacrifice tasty food in exchange for their health. My goal is to make meals so delicious that no one has to sacrifice anything but sickness and disease, which is a sacrifice most are willing to make.

I have developed a comprehensive program that includes a balanced plant-based approach accompanied by a comprehensive coaching program that enhances the experience and encourages success both in the office and online.

I have lots of dinner parties at out home and people forget that they are not eating meat and they love it. I have frequently been asked if I would write a cookbook.

I started writing a cookbook about 10 years ago, and it is still not complete. As inspiration, my "favorite husband" took some of my recipes and put them in a book and presented to me the only printed copy of Dr. Helen's Everyday Gourmet as a Christmas present some 8 years ago. You see why he's my favorite? Ok, so he is my only one, but I like saying that. At any rate, he presented my copy of my recipes to me to inspire me to write my book. Did I mention that was 8 years ago? It is still nicely displayed in my kitchen.

That book is now being transformed into a full cookbook of plant-based foods that help maintain this plant-based lifestyle even after the **Reverse it!** jumpstart is over. It has incredibly delicious and interesting food recipes to help support this plant-based lifestyle for ongoing prevention of chronic diseases. It is called "**The Genesis Plan**." I can't wait to finish it. I have done more research and have had more experiences on reversing type 2 diabetes since I started the book 10 years ago. Some things are worth the wait.

In medical school, we were taught that type 2 diabetes was a chronic disease with inevitable complications if fasting blood glucose levels were not controlled. Even with the best control and even with our best efforts, the best we could ever hope for was to delay the inevitable problems that were likely to arise over time.

I didn't learn that type 2 diabetes could actually be reversed until I started treating patients with diabetes for myself. I experienced it up close and personal.

This is contrary to the prevailing thought that type 2 diabetes is a lifelong disease with no cure, but this is not the case.

As a matter of fact, a pilot study published in Preventive Medicine in 1999 found that when significant dietary changes of low fat, vegetarian foods were consumed, 66% of the patients with diabetes in the study were able to reduce or eliminate their diabetic medications within 12 weeks (10). Since that time, even more studies have confirmed that type 2 diabetes is, indeed, reversible (11, 12, 16, 17, 18, 20).

Twelve weeks is spectacular to reverse type 2 diabetes, but I discovered an even faster approach by starting with a detoxification program. Our program involves juicing and raw, non GMO fruits, vegetables, nuts and seeds to accelerate the process.

I created and developed the detoxification plan to provide the blueprint to jumpstart reversing type 2 diabetes and other chronic diseases like lupus (13), hypertension, heart disease (14, 15), and of course, obesity (16, 17, 19).

I have many patients that come into my office complaining about the struggles they have with type 2 diabetes. They complain about the medications and its side effects, the finger pricks, the complications, and the pain. I can empathize with their experience because I have been intimately associated with this unfortunate chronic health challenge.

It is lamentable that most people have no idea that reversing type 2 diabetes is even possible. When I mention it to my patients, they are often awestruck by the possibility. Even those who suspect reversal as a possibility have no clue as to how to accomplish such a seemingly major feat.

But type 2 diabetes is nothing more than a challenge. It can be overcome. Using the word "challenge" assigns a different meaning and promotes a feeling of hope and not despair. When the word "challenge" is used, it suggests that a transformation is possible. It is.

Transformation is possible. Type 2 diabetes can be reversed. It is not only possible, but countless studies have now proven it to be the case (10, 11, 12, 13, 14, 15, 16, 17, 18, 19, 20). Here is just one example.

My patient DB

DB was referred to my office complaining of fatigue, sleep disturbance, and low back pain. She was diabetic with heart disease, high cholesterol, diabetic peripheral neuropathy, and had fallen several times. She was using a walker for support due to diabetic peripheral neuropathy.

She was on three medications for blood pressure, one for chest pain, one anti-coagulant, two oral hypoglycemics and both long acting and short acting insulin.

Her weight was 207 lbs with a BMI of 35.53, HbA1c 6.0%, FBS 151 (on 3 different medications). She had renal insufficiency with an elevated creatinine. Her blood pressure was maintained, but on three different drugs.

We started her on our detoxification program that included juicing, smoothies, and balanced raw meals and placed her on a light walking plan of 30 minutes per day at least 3 times per week. We gave her the tools to avoid hypoglycemia. Her FBS rapidly decreased in the first few weeks and she lost 10 pounds in 30 days. Her energy level rapidly increased. Her blood pressure normalized on no blood pressure medications so her doctor discontinued them altogether.

Within 3 months, she was 183 lbs (a loss of 24 lbs) with a BMI of 31 and when we checked her HbA1c at 3 months, it was 5.6% (see Table 1).

Our goal was only to control her diabetes, but she had the fortunate side effect of weight loss, improved energy, normalization of blood pressure and decreased risk of cardiovascular disease. The patient was pleased to continue her plant-based lifestyle even when she was lost to follow up.

Table 1

DAY	WEIGHT (LBS)	BMI
1	207.00	36
30	197.00	34
60	190.00	33
90	183.00	31
120	174.00	30
150	168.00	29

DB'S SIDE EFFECT - WEIGHT LOSS

She admits that she did not continue with the program explicitedly, but she continued some of the recipes we recommended. Several months had elapsed when we finally caught up with her. It was 9 months later, and we were pleased that she was able to maintain a stable lowered BP. Her HbA1c remained at 5.6%. Weight was well-controlled at 156.2 (ideal body 108-132 lbs) and BMI was 26.61.

All this, without restarting insulin and only one blood pressure medication. DB reported a continued increase in energy and an overall feeling of well-being. She hadn't fully maintained the program, but reported that she restarted her new lifestyle because she felt much better on plant-based foods than on animal-based foods.

Her average weight loss was 2 pounds per week or 8 pounds per month (see Figure 1). Her BMI steadily decreased (see Figure 2). The decrease in BMI and weight loss were considerable, but the best part is her increase in insulin sensitivity.

Her insulin level started at 19.7 at the beginning of our program and decreased to 4.84 in 3 months. All of that excess insulin at the onset of our program was used to get her fasting blood sugar to 107. We were able to increase her insulin sensitivity to 4.84 and produced a fasting blood sugar of 99 on no hypoglycemic medications. Less insulin leads to less fat storage since insulin is a fat storage hormone.

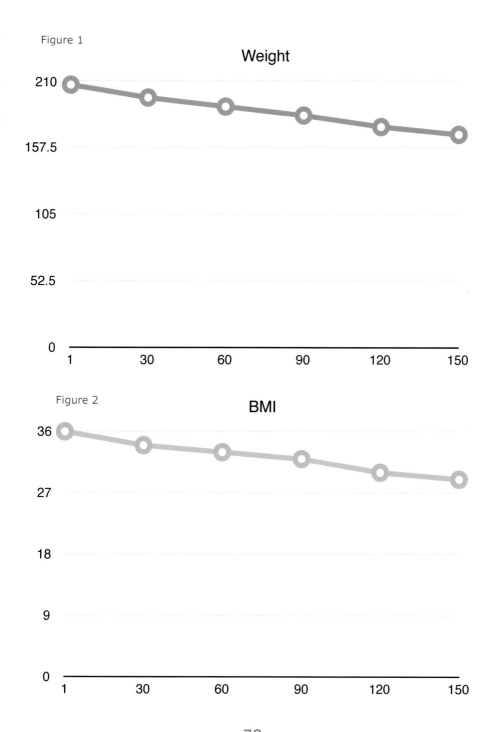

Figure 1

Weight

Figure 2

BMI

Chapter 6

Why Detox?

Toxins are found everywhere. They are in everything from the air we breathe, the paint on the walls, the carpet we walk on, the water we drink, the pesticides in our food, the shower gels, soaps, lotions and deodorants we put on our bodies to the processed foods we consume. These substances build up in our tissues, organs, blood and lymphatic system and lead to fatigue and metabolic disturbances.

The primary process of detoxification occurs in the liver—the main detoxifying organ. Its job is to cleanse toxins and waste products from the blood. In the process, it will separate out the nutrients that are necessary for the body to function correctly. It also activates and regulates many essential hormones. This is literally just of few of the hundreds of tasks that the liver performs on a daily basis.

In type 2 diabetes, one of the major problems is an inability to lose weight. This is due to insulin resistance, which inhibits the effectiveness of fat burning hormones, while also increasing appetite and carbohydrate cravings.

Besides, most, if not all, people with type 2 diabetes have a fatty liver. A fatty liver indicates that the liver is unable to properly burn fat leading to a slower metabolism.

The liver becomes fatty because of an increase in the wrong type of carbohydrates like white flour, sugar, pasta, bread, etc., and the wrong kind of fats. When these foods are consumed in excess, the liver can not adequately metabolize them. It can, however, convert excess carbohydrates to fat and can use the wrong fats to store in the liver. This leads to non-alcoholic fatty liver disease (NAFLD).

NAFLD is related to insulin resistance. The treatment for NAFLD is weight loss. However, it becomes a catch 22 when there is insulin resistance leading to increasingly elevated levels of insulin, which worsens fat storage (21, 22, 23).

Detoxification is a great way to interrupt this vicious cycle while encouraging weight loss and improving insulin sensitivity simultaneously. This will lead to better overall health of the liver.

To obtain and maintain optimum health, we must be able to eliminate waste so that it is not allowed to reaccumulate and recirculate in our bodies and wreak havoc on the DNA of our cells leading to organ damage especially in the pancreas and liver.

Most people don't understand that it is necessary to detoxify to clean out our bodies. We clean everything else like our cars, houses, desks, and refrigerators, but fail to clean our bodies.

When toxins deposit into the tissues of the body, imbalances occur that can manifest into many health-related challenges. This can lead to blurred vision, memory loss, central nervous system disorders, unexplained weight gain, fatigue, insomnia, skin problems, varicose veins, heart problems, diabetes, low testosterone in men, joint inflammation and stiffness, acid reflux and GERD, increased risk of certain cancers such as breast and colon, back pain, and IBS just to name a few.

Detoxification is a great way to restart the metabolic thermostat and reduce food cravings by stabilizing sugar levels.

Elimination of toxins reduces inflammation, and transitions the body from a disease-prone acidic state to a disease-fighting alkaline state.

Chapter 7

Detoxification

When food enters the mouth and moves through

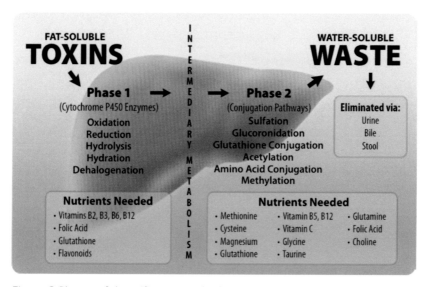

Figure 3 Phases of detoxification in the liver

the digestive system, the food is broken down into smaller particles that then enter the blood and then the liver for filtration. The liver extracts nutrients to be used by the body from the waste products or toxins that will ultimately be removed from the body. It is a constant event for the liver.

Removing toxic substances from the body creates elements that can be more dangerous than the original toxin. Therefore, the liver must safely remove toxins from the blood through 2 separate phases of detoxification. Through a series of steps, the waste products are converted to less toxic substances to be either carried out in the bile into the small intestines and subsequently the stool, or it will be carried by the blood into the kidneys and finally into the urine. These 2 processes are called Phase 1 and Phase 2 detoxification of the liver.

It is imperative that both phase 1 and phase 2 of detoxification be balanced with the proper nutrition at each stage. If the nutrients are out of balance, the intermediate metabolites of the first phase of detoxification, being more toxic than the original substance, will recirculate in the blood as free radicals and damage the DNA of the cells and ultimately lead to disease.

When the phases are in balance, and the proper nutrients are provided, phase 2 detoxification will continue the processing of waste and be eliminated through the stool or the urine.

Literally, every drug consumed, every artificial chemical that enters the body, every pesticide or its residue on our food and every hormone is metabolized or broken down by enzyme pathways in the liver cells.

The substances enter the body as fat-soluble substances that are not eliminated in the body because they can only be dissolved in oily or fatty solutions and not water. They have a high affinity for fatty tissues and the membranes or coverings of the cells of the body. It is for this reason that toxins can be stored in fat for many years and is only released during times of stress, exercise or fasting. The cellulite you see is a result of this toxic storage.

When the toxins are released, symptoms of detoxification may occur including headaches, memory disturbances, abdominal pain, fatigue, nausea, dizziness, and palpitations. Sugar cravings may also occur.

These fat-soluble substances must, therefore, be transformed into water-soluble materials and eliminated by the body in the stool or urine through a series of enzymes referred to as the cytochrome P450 system.

This system of enzymes is housed in the cells of the liver called hepatocytes. During this process, many free radicals are produced and can subsequently damage the liver, if excessive. Antioxidants are necessary to protect the liver from these toxic free radicals (see Table 2).

Table 2

Nutrient	Purpose	Foods
Arginine	Needed to detoxify ammonia, which is a waste product of protein metabolism	It is found in legumes, seeds, walnuts and wheat germ
Antioxidants	Needed to neutralize free radicals	Raw juices, apple, pear, carrots, dandelion, chorella, spirulina, fresh fruits
Methionine	Essential for detoxification	Legumes, garlic, onions, seeds (also found in eggs, fish, meat, but these carry their own toxins)
Essential fatty acids	Required for healthy membrane and healthy liver function	Avocado, fresh raw nuts, seeds, spinach, green beans and peas, eggplant, flax seeds, evening primrose
Glutathione	Super antioxidant produced in the liver where it detoxifies harmful substances to be excreted in the bile. It is important in phase 1 and phase 2 of detoxification	Mostly made from its precursors cysteine, glycine and glutamate, but also found in small amounts in asparagus, avocado, spinach, okra, broccoli, cantaloupe, tomato, carrot, grapefruit (others)
Alpha-lipoic acid (ALA)	Powerful antioxidant and is a recycler of both Vitamin E and Vitamin C. Stimulates the production of glutathione and in the absorption of CoQ10. Neutralizes free radicals	Spinach, broccoli potatoes, brewer's yeast, organ meats (but these contain major toxins)
Milk thistle (Silymarin)	Guards the liver against oxidative damage from phase 1 detoxification. Promotes the growth of new liver cells. Also increases levels of glutathione, superoxide dismutase and catalase.	Turmeric root, coriander seeds, cilantro, dark grapes, beet greens, berries, supplements

This list is not exhaustive

Pesticides, for instance, can significantly disrupt this pathway and cause overactivity of this P450 system producing very high levels of free radicals. The result is damage to the DNA of the cells of the body leading to disease.

A few of the nutrients needed for proper detoxification are included in the table.

Depending on the number of toxins found in the body and the speed of detoxification, symptoms may occur. It is essential to recognize them as part of the process and not as an actual illness.

Some of the symptoms of detoxification include nausea, headaches, muscle aches, low-grade fever, thirst, rashes, constipation, extreme food cravings, gas, bloating, irritability, diarrhea, and vomiting. Intractable vomiting requires further investigation by your doctor.

These symptoms are transient and should slow down within the first 1-2 weeks. If symptoms extend beyond this time, you may be detoxing too quickly. If this occurs, add in some cooked vegetables or vegetable broths or soups and restart once symptoms have dissipated. Be sure to discuss with your doctor.

It is also imperative to drink purified water regularly throughout the day. My goal is to drink about six 16 oz juices every 2-2.5 hours daily. After the first 10 days, begin eating raw foods and eat to fullness. Drink pure water between juices and meals to aid in flushing the toxins from the body. A limited amount of unsweetened herbal teas are permitted. You will urinate a lot. You are releasing toxins. With that in mind, let's get started!

Let's Get Started!

Eden Good

Water

Refreshing and Detoxifying Water with Lemon

Drink 16-32 oz of water with fresh lemon each morning upon rising. It will refresh you, begin digestion and hydrate you where it really counts.

Instructions

I am not accustomed to putting the fruits and vegetables in the hopper in any particular order unless there is some fruit like a very ripe pear. If my pear is very soft, I will use a stronger fruit or vegetable to push it through the hopper. I prefer to have the fruit a little firmer and save the more ripe fruit for smoothies. If a fruit is ripe before I am ready to use it, I will usually wash and dry the fruit thoroughly and then freeze so that they are ready for use when I am.

Notes and Favorites

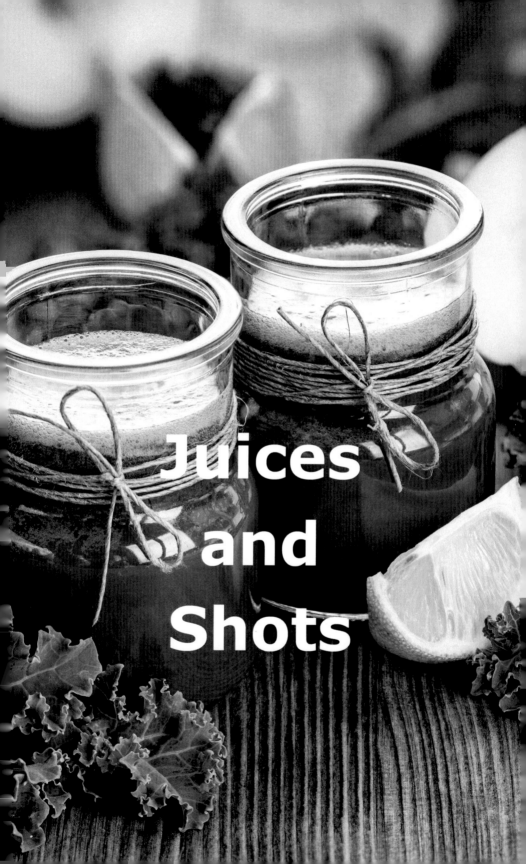

Juices
and
Shots

Get Me Started!

5 c spinach
1 large cucumber
2 pears
1 carrot
1 celery stalk
½ lemon, unpeeled
1 inch fresh ginger

PS I usually do a 30-day cleanse in January, but I decided to do it in November because I really wanted to test the recipes again. I enjoyed the flavors. It may require straining if the pears are soft. The taste is delicious! Enjoy!

Green Beet

2 large kale leaves
1 apple
1 orange, peeled
½ beet
1 celery stick
½ lemon
1 inch fresh ginger

PS This is a beautiful juice for detoxification. It supports both phases of detoxification by providing antioxidants necessary for the liver to process and eliminate. It is also quite tasty. Enjoy!

Kick Some Kale

1 bunch of kale (include stems)
2 cucumbers (unpeeled)
½ c mint
Juice of ½ lemon
½ c pineapple
¼ inch fresh ginger (unpeeled)
Dash of cayenne pepper

PS I am sipping on this one as I write. It is dinner time, and I thought this would be a great choice, and I was right. Enjoy!

Red Runner

2 Roma tomatoes
2 cucumbers
1 garlic clove
1 c cilantro

1 shallot or ¼ c sweet onion
Juice of 1 lime
Dash of cayenne pepper

PS The Red Runner is one of the easiest to make
and is a wonderful dinner juice. The cayenne
pepper gives it a nice kick while it increases
circulation. Enjoy!

Italian Sipper

2 c kale, stems included
2 Roma tomatoes
2 red bell peppers
1 garlic clove
¼ c fresh basil leaves
Pinch of cayenne pepper

PS I used lots of basil in this one because I love
Italian flavors. I also used more than a pinch of
cayenne because I like spicy food. I think I got
that from my mom. Enjoy!

The Beet Goes On

½ large beet
2 carrots
1 apple (green)
½ fresh ginger

PS Beets are highly nutritious and are excellent for cardiovascular and blood vessel health. Men need to know that it helps with erections. It is an excellent source of glycine betaine that lowers homocysteine levels leading to a lower incidence of clot formation in the blood. High levels of homocysteine promotes coronary heart disease, stroke, and peripheral vascular disease. Beets are an excellent vasodilator and contains very high amounts of Nitric oxide, just call it Viagra minus the possible sudden vision loss. Lol! Enjoy!

The Greenery

5 kale leaves
1 cucumber
2 handfuls of spinach
1 green apple
1 celery stalk
1 lime, peeled

PS There are plenty of antioxidants in this juice.
Antioxidants are needed for phase 1 detoxification
to neutralize the intermediate metabolites. Enjoy!

Partial To Parsley

2 cucumbers
1 c fresh Italian or curly parsley
1 pear
1 fennel bulb
¼ mint leaves

PS Fennel is available in bulb, leaf, seed and stalk forms.
I like to add fennel leaf and bulb to salads, and I using
the seeds to mimic a sausage flavor along with sage
and smoked paprika (more on this in the Genesis Plan).
I learned that from the apron strings of my mom. Enjoy!

Roman Beet

1 head romaine lettuce
1 large beet
1 cucumber
5 carrots
1 inch fresh ginger

The Eye Opener

5 large carrots
1 head of romaine lettuce
2 oranges

PS Oranges are an excellent source of Vitamin C and phytochemicals that scavenge free radicals and serve as immune system modulators. They also contain beta-carotene, zeaxanthin, and lutein that are essential for healthy eyesight. They contain potassium that helps to control blood pressure and heart rate. There are many other nutrients as well. Enjoy!

Kale-Aboration

4 kale leaves
4 oranges
6 tangerines
1 fennel stem
2 celery stalks
Juice of 2 limes
½ inch fresh ginger

Vision

2 c spinach
5 carrots
1 orange
1 inch fresh ginger
5 mint sprigs

Anti-Flam

4 sweet potatoes
8 carrots
2 Gala or Fuji apples
2 cucumbers

1 inch fresh ginger
½ t turmeric (stir in)

Bringing In The Greens

2 c spinach
2 c kale
1 c collards
2 celery stalks
½ cucumber
2 green apples
½ c fresh mint
Juice of ½ lemon
½-1 inch fresh ginger (optional)

PS Spinach is an excellent source of many vitamins and minerals. It contains high amounts of carotenoids such as zeaxanthin that protects against age-related macular disease in older adults. It is rich with folic acid that prevents neural tube defects in newborns. Its iron content protects against anemia. It contains many minerals including potassium, magnesium, copper, zinc, and manganese that are all necessary for proper function of the body.

Spinach is also a rich source for vitamins such as vitamin C, a powerful antioxidant, that helps the body resist infection and scavenge free radicals that can damage the DNA of individual cells.

It also contains vitamin K that plays a vital roll in bone strengthening and limiting neuronal damage in the brain. Its content of vitamin A is essential for night vision. It has multiple B vitamins, It is required at all stages of life from newborn to the aged. It is fabulous for both phases of detoxification. Enjoy!

I'm Kale'n It

5 kale leaves
1 green apple, cored and quartered
½ cucumber
2 celery stalks
1 lime, halved
1 inch fresh ginger

Redicious

5 kales leaves
4 romaine leaves
4 carrots
1 medium beet
2 celery stalks
¼ fresh parsley
1 inch fresh ginger

C-Shot

1 orange, peeled
1 lime, peeled
2 inches fresh ginger

Heavy Metal Buster Shot

2 limes
1 handful fresh cilantro
½ inch fresh ginger

Keep It Movin' Shot

½ beet
1 lemon, peeled
½ inch fresh ginger
dash of cayenne pepper

Shot to Kill

2 inches fresh ginger
2 T coconut water
juice of ½ lemon
½ t apple cider vinegar (with the mother)
1 turmeric finger or ¼ t ground turmeric
Pinch of black pepper

Gingered Lemon Shot

2 inches fresh ginger
juice of 1 lemon
dash of cayenne pepper

Allergy Bust Shot

½ c fresh pineapple
1 t bee pollen
juice of 1 lemon
1 drop peppermint oil
1 drop lavender oil
¼ c water

Puttin' Out The Fire

1 Turmeric finger
2 inches fresh ginger
dash of black pepper
1 lemon
¼ c water

PS Use a blender to get these shots

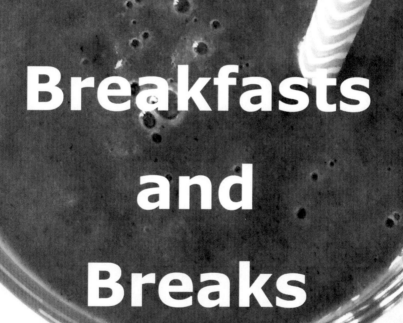

Breakfasts
and
Breaks

Instructions

Place all ingredients in a high-speed blender and blend until smooth. If you do not have a high-speed blender, chop your vegetables smaller and blend for longer.

*Nuts are optional and can be used for added protein or nuts can be replaced with a high quality plant-based protein powder in your smoothies.

Healing Anti-Aging Berry Blast

5 c red chard
2 c frozen mixed berries or blueberries
1 c coconut water
1 c pomegranate juice
1 c filtered water
1 t baobab powder (optional)
2 T chia seeds

Healing Cherry Smoothie

5 c red chard, packed
½ avocado
2 c organic sweet cherries
1/4 c raw cashews
3 c water
3 T chia seeds
1 t baobab powder (optional)
1 c ice (optional)

Healing Chocolana Smoothie

2 ripe organic bananas

5 c fresh kale

1 c raw cashews

½ avocado

2 T cacao

1 T maca

1 T flax seeds

4 c water

1 c ice

cacao nibs (optional garnish)

PS Cashews are delicious, slightly sweet, but high in calories. One cup is about 600 calories, so be careful. I love them for their taste, but also because they help to lower LDL cholesterol (the bad one) and increase HDL cholesterol (the good one). Enjoy!

Healing Orange Mango Magic

3 c spinach
3 c kale, stems removed if using a regular blender
2 large seeded oranges, peeled
2 carrots
1 t orange zest
1 c frozen mango
1 c filtered water
2 c coconut water
¼ c flaxseeds
1 c ice (optional)

Healing Give It A Rest Smoothie

5 c fresh kale
2 c fresh frozen blueberries
3 c water
½ avocado
½ t lavender flowers if dried (or 1 t if fresh depending on your taste, 1-2 drops of lavender oil is also nice)

1 lemon, juiced
1 T local honey, if desired

Healing Inflammation Buster Upper Smoothie

6 c spinach
2 fingers of fresh turmeric, washed, peeled
1 inch fresh organic ginger, washed, peeled
⅛ t ground coriander
⅛ t ground cardamom
1 t vanilla extract (the real kind)
3 c water
1-2 pitted Medjool dates, optional
¼ c flax seeds
1 c ice
dash of black pepper

Healing With Parental Discretion Advisement Smoothie

4 c spinach

1 t maca powder

½ medium avocado

1 T cacao powder

1 ripe organic banana

1-2 Medjool dates, pitted (optional)

3 c water

¼ c chia seeds

1 c ice

Healing Mango-Banana Smoothie

6 c fresh kale

½ ripe organic banana

1 ripe mango

2 c water

1 c ice

Healing Pineapple Tangerine Cream Smoothie

2 handfuls of fresh kale (about 5-6 c)
3 tangerines, peeled
1 cup fresh pineapple
¼ - ½ avocado
3 T chia seeds
4 c water
1 c ice

Healing Fan of the Beet!

2 heaping handfuls of spinach (about 6 cups)
½ medium beet
½ c frozen pineapple
1 orange
1 inch of orange skin (zest)
1 c water
1 c ice

Healing Mango Orange Smoothie

6 c fresh spinach
1 c coconut water
1 c water
1 orange (pith removed)
½ t orange zest (optional)
1 c frozen mango
2 T chia seeds
4-6 ice cubes if needed

Healing Pina Grenada Smoothie

6 c fresh spinach
1 c frozen pineapple
2 c water
1 c coconut water
1 t coconut extract
1 T flax seeds
1 c ice

Healing Pineapple Gingered Smoothie

5-6 c fresh kale

2 pineapple spears

1 handful of almonds

2 inches fresh ginger (more if you like ginger)

2 T flaxseeds

3 c water

1 c ice

Healing Power Up! Smoothie

3 c spinach

3 c kale

2 c frozen mango

3 c water

1 in fresh ginger peeled

½ c pumpkin seeds

Juice of 1 lemon plus 1 t grated zest

3 dates pitted, optional

2 T flaxseeds

Ice (optional)

Healing Blueberry Beet Smoothie

3 c swiss chard, red
½ beet
1 pint blueberries
1 ripe organic banana
handful of almonds
2-3 dates, optional
1 T spirulina
1 c water
1 c iceHealing Tropical Smoothie

6 c kale

1 kiwi, peeled

1 c pineapple chunks

1-inch fresh ginger

1 mango, peeled

2 T chia seeds

2 c water

1 c ice

Healing Ginger Beet Smoothie

½ beet
1 apple, cored
1-inch ginger
½ lemon juice
2 carrots
1 c water
2 c ice
1 T chia seeds

Healing Strawberry Banana Mango Smoothie

6 c kale
1 ripe organic banana
1 c strawberries, washed with tops on
1 mango, peeled
1 T flaxseeds
1 c water
handful of almonds
1 c ice

Healing Blueberry Beet Banana Smoothie

3 c Swiss chard, red
½ beet
1 pint blueberries
½ ripe organic banana
handful of almonds
1 c water
1 c ice

Healing Strawberry Banana Cream Smoothie

5-6 c greens
2 c strawberries with the tops
½ ripe organic banana
1 T flaxseeds
¼ c cashew
3 c water
juice of 1 lemon
1 c ice

Healing Triple C Smoothie

6 c kale
½ cantaloupe
1 medium carrot
1 c almonds
1 t cinnamon
1-inch fresh ginger
3 c water
1 c ice

Healing Berry Tropical Smoothie

6 c kale
1 c fresh or frozen strawberries, tops on
1 c fresh or frozen blueberries
1-inch fresh ginger
1 mango, peeled
1 T spirulina
2 T chia seeds
2 c water
1 c ice

Healing Berry Beet Smoothie (2)

5-6 c kale
½ large beet
½ ripe organic banana
1 pint blueberries
1 handful of almonds
1 T flaxseeds
juice of ½ lemon
2 c water
1 c ice

Healing Pitaya Bowl

2 packets frozen unsweetened pitaya puree (3.5 oz)
1 ripe organic banana
1 t maca powder
1 t chia seeds
¼ c water or coconut water for blending
toppings
¼ c blueberries
¼ c raw cashews
¼ c unsweetened granola
¼ c mango, cubed

PS In a blender, add pitaya puree, date, banana, maca powder, chia seeds and coconut water. Blend until the mixture is smooth, thick and creamy. Pour into a bowl. Top with mango, granola, blueberries and cashews in sections or all on top. You can really arrange it any way you like. See recipe for granola in the snack section. Enjoy!

Healing Citrus Bowl

2 kiwi, sliced
1 pint blueberries
1 grapefruit, sliced
2 oranges, sliced
1 mango, pitted and sliced

PS Arrange fruit on a platter and enjoy. No need to add any sugar. Allow the natural sweetness of the fruit to tantalize your tastebuds. Have as a breakfast salad or an anytime snack. Enjoy!

Healing Acai Bowl

2 packets unsweetened frozen acai purée (4oz)
(found in frozen fruit section)
1 medium organic banana, cut in ½
2 T flaxseeds
toppings
1 persimmon (can replace with other fruit)
¼ c coconut flakes
¼ c cashews
¼ c blueberries
¼ c unsweetened granola

PS Run Acai packets under hot water to loosen from the packet and blend with ½ banana and honey, stopping to stir to break up the mixture as needed. It should be thick. Transfer to a bowl and top with the remaining banana, blueberries, persimmon, and low sugar granola (if desired). Remember presentation is key. Enjoy!

Healing Overnight Oats

½ organic banana
½ c gluten-free oats
1 c almond milk

1 t vanilla
1 T flaxseeds
1 T chia seeds
1 c strawberries (save 2-4 for topping)
Almonds for garnish

PS Mix together banana, strawberries (saving a few for topping), vanilla, milk and lemon in a blender to combine well. Fill 6-8 oz mason jar or cup with 1/2 oats. Pour over strawberry cream mixture, stir and refrigerate overnight or at least an hour. After all the strawberry cream soaks in add flaxseeds, chia seeds, strawberries, and almonds. Enjoy!

Healing Fruit Casserole

2 Granny Smith apples sliced
1 clamshell of strawberries
1 pint of blueberries

PS Presentation is everything. It can mean the difference between wanting to eat something and leaving it along. Arrange the apple slices around the edge of a platter. Next, layer in the strawberries. Lastly, place the blueberries in the center. Consume it as a breakfast salad or anytime snack. Enjoy!

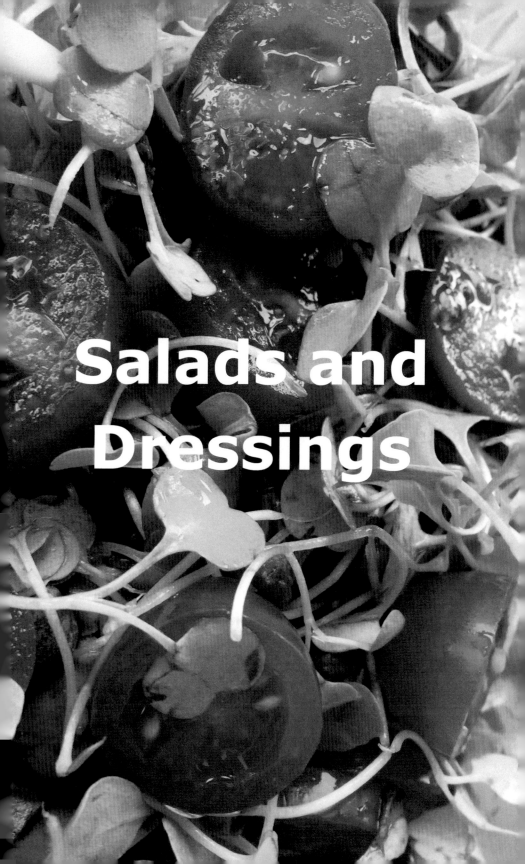

Salads and Dressings

Greens are a natural detoxifier and are gentle enough to consume every day. There are different types of greens including kale, swiss chard, spinach, arugula, frisée, radicchio, butter lettuce, romaine, green leaf, dandelion, etc. The leaves of these greens are much more nutritious than iceberg lettuce which is just a water source and not recommended.

Using greens, you will have a great source of vitamin A for vision, Vitamin C for a healthy immune system, Magnesium that relaxes muscles and maintains blood pressure as well as Folate and Iron to provide healthy blood.

They are amenable to different additions including the typical tomatoes and cucumbers, but you can get creative by adding different raw vegetables that boost the flavor and interest of your salads. Feel free to add raw nuts, raw seeds, fresh fruits, and other vegetables for a clean, crisp taste.

Salad dressings are easy to make and frankly, not necessary to buy. By making your own, you avoid all the unnecessary additives and preservatives that increase the size of your waistline. You can be as creative as you like. You will know what is in it what you create. Your homemade salad dressings will add so much to an already inviting meal. Enjoy!

Healing Citrus Salad

1 clamshell of mixed greens
1 c cherry tomatoes
1 c cucumber, diced
½ c mandarin oranges
½ c raw almonds

PS Consider Healing Ginger-Orange Dressing. Assemble washed and dried ingredients. Make the dressing by placing all items into a food processor. Adjust taste to your liking if needed. Enjoy!

Healing Pineapple Beet Salad

1 large beet, shredded
¼ c fresh pineapple, chopped (save juice)
½ T minced ginger
1 T orange zest
2 T pine nuts (optional)

PS Shred beets and pineapple in a bowl and add grated ginger then orange zest. Use simple dressing to toss in with the beets. Sprinkle pine nuts. Serve cold. Enjoy!

Healing All In Salad

15 oz organic chickpeas
3 cups raw kale (~3 large leaves, loosely packed)
¼ c purple cabbage, thinly sliced
12 fresh Brussels sprouts, thinly sliced
½ c green leaf lettuce, sliced
6 oz black olives, sliced
¼ thinly sliced red onion

PS Toss all salad ingredients together and put aside. Sprinkle Dulse flakes on top particularly if there is hypothyroid disease or slowed metabolism. Choose your favorite dressing. Enjoy!

Healing Curry Chick'n Salad in Collard Wrap

1 c walnuts, soaked overnight
½ tsp cumin
1 tsp chick'n seasoning

½ t turmeric

1 t nutritional yeast flakes

½ t ground garlic

½ onion, chopped

¼ c dried cranberries

1 ripe avocado, mashed

PS Drain and rinse walnuts. In a food processor, pulse walnuts to desired consistency. Add avocado and mix well with fresh lime. Add dry ingredients except for cranberries. Stir together well. Toss in cranberries. Use a collard, cabbage or kale leaf to wrap. Enjoy!

Healing Chickun' Salad

2 c soaked walnuts

1 celery stick sliced

⅓ sweet onion

1 T nutritional yeast flakes

1 t onion powder

1 t dried oregano

½ t turmeric

2 T water (as needed to get the mixture going)

salt to taste, if needed

PS Soaking the walnuts overnight is the longest part of this recipe. Whenever I make this, I want to eat more of it. It is so worth it. Soak on! Soak walnuts 8 hours or overnight. Rinse and drain and pulse in high-speed blender or food processor until crumbly. Add onion and continue to pulse. Mix in nutritional yeast, onion powder, oregano and turmeric. Add a little water to make into a slightly creamy mixture (instead of mayo). Lastly, stir in sliced celery. Enjoy!

Healing Corn and Kale Salad

5 ears nonGMO corn, cut off the cob, (see note)
1 c cherry tomatoes (about 20)
2 c kale, sliced into small, bite-sized pieces
1 can black olives, sliced
1 juicy lime
1 T oregano
1 T nutritional yeast flakes
½ c fresh cilantro, chopped

PS Wash tomatoes and cut in half. Cut corn off the cob into a bowl. Toss in chopped kale and sliced olives. Season with oregano, nutritional yeast flakes, and cilantro. Squeeze fresh lime juice on top. Use only organic, non-GMO corn. If you are challenged with candida, please choose another recipe.

Healing Kimchi

1 red cabbage, sliced thinly
3 garlic cloves, grated
1 small onion sliced
1 T smoked paprika
1 t cayenne pepper
2 T sea salt
3 T ACV
½ c purified or distilled water

PS Place all solid ingredients into a large bowl and sprinkle with salt. Massage the cabbage to soften. Add water and ACV. Prepare mason jars by placing in boiling water for 10 minutes (tops included). Once hot, remove from pot and put right side up. This process will prevent unwanted bacterial growth. Now, separate into mason jars and top it. Allow to sit in a warm place 1-5 days and shake a few times every day. Refrigerate. Enjoy!

Healing mixed Greens Salad

1 small clamshell of mixed greens, washed and dried
1 large cucumber
1 red pepper, sliced
4 radishes, halved and then sliced
1 c cherry tomatoes, sliced in half
1 large tomato, sliced
1 c black olives
½ medium red onion, sliced

PS Layer each ingredient on each level so that each bite has a mixture of all of the yummy goodness. Enjoy!

Healing Citrus and Sumac Salad

1 5 oz clamshell of mixed spinach and arugula
½ small red onion, thinly sliced
½ c fresh basil
2 oranges with membranes removed

3 T flaxseeds
½ c raw almonds, sliced or whole

PS Start with ½ of the greens and layer in your salad bowl followed by ½ the red onions, basil, oranges, flaxseeds, and almonds. Repeat a second layer. Sprinkle sumac salad dressing (see Sumac dressing recipe) or any other favorite dressing. Enjoy!

Healing Avocado Salad

1 small clamshell of arugula
1 cucumber, thinly sliced
3 ripe avocados, thinly slice 2 ½ of them and save the last half for dressing
1 c fresh cilantro leaves coarsely chopped, saving some whole
1 t nigella seeds
2 green chilis, seeded and thinly sliced at an angle
  (seeded jalapeño can work for a little kick)
1 garlic clove
1 T fresh lime juice
1 T amino acids
1 T ACV

PS Combine arugula, cucumber, avocado, cilantro, and nigella seeds. In a high-speed blender, combine ½ avocado, garlic, green chilis, lime juice, amino acids, and ACV and mix to form a nice thick green dressing. For a thinner consistency, add a little water. Pour over salad. Enjoy!

Healing Kale Avocado Salad

1 bunch fresh kale, coarsely chopped
½ red onion, chopped
¼ c cherry tomatoes, sliced
2 avocados, mashed
2 T nutritional yeast flakes
2 t smoked paprika
1 t dried oregano
juice of 1 lemon
salt to taste
⅛ t cayenne pepper, optional

PS In a large container, mash avocado and squeeze fresh lemon over it. Add onion, nutritional yeast, paprika, oregano, and salt to taste and combine to mix well. Fold in tomatoes and stir in kale to blend well. Add cayenne pepper, if using. Adjust seasoning as needed. Enjoy!

Healing Chopped Cucumber Avocado Salad

1 cucumber, cubed
1 avocado, cubed
½ pint of grape tomatoes, halved
1 can of black olives
2 T fresh cilantro
½ lime, juiced
⅛ c walnuts
1 t garlic powder
1 t oregano
1 t amino acid

PS Cut all vegetables and place in a medium bowl. Sprinkle with seasonings and toss together. Add walnuts and stir. Serve cold. Enjoy!

Healing Corn Avocado Salad

2 ears of fresh nonGMO corn on the cob
½ ripe avocado
juice of 1 lemon
6 cherry tomatoes, diced
2 T nutritional yeast flakes
1 t smoked paprika
¼ c chopped cilantro
⅛ t cayenne pepper
salt to taste

PS Mash avocado with juice of 1 lemon, salt, paprika, oregano and 1T water if needed. Mix with corn and adjust seasoning as needed. Enjoy!

Healing Vegetable Korma

½ head cauliflower, broken into bite-size pieces
2 carrots, cut on diagonal
2 medium tomatoes
3 T chopped red onion
2 inches ginger
1 small garlic clove
½ teaspoon turmeric powder
½ teaspoon chili powder
½ teaspoon mustard seed
½ teaspoon cumin seeds
1 T cilantro leaves (plus more for garnish)
3 T dried grated young coconut slices
1 T garam masala
2 dried red chilies
2 t coriander seeds
¼ t fenugreek seeds
4 T water (or to desired consistency 1 T at a time)
juice of ½ lime
salt to taste, optional

PS Break cauliflower into small, bite-sized pieces.
Slice carrots on the diagonal and toss with
cauliflower. Set aside. In a high-speed blender, add
all the other ingredients except lime and cashews

and either place Vitamix on "hot soups" or blend until smooth about 5 minutes. Toss into cauliflower and carrots and coat well. Squeeze the juice of ½ lime over mixture, salt to taste and fold in cashews when ready to eat to keep the cashews crisp. Garnish with fresh cilantro. Enjoy!

Healing Kale Salad in Coconut Wrap

1 bunch fresh kale, hard stems removed
¼ c nutritional yeast flakes
1 soft avocado
1 lime, juiced
2 T smoked paprika
¼ c red onions, diced
salt to taste

PS Chop kale to bite-sized pieces removing hard, woody stems. Add nutritional yeast flakes, smoked paprika, lime, onion and avocado, and massage into kale. Generously spoon mixture into store-bought coconut wraps. You may substitute for seaweed wrap/nori wrap for a meaty taste. Enjoy!

Healing Asian Wraps

10 small or 5 small rice paper sheets
2 c fresh spinach
1 small head romaine lettuce
1 large carrot, julienned or cut into strips
1 small cucumber, julienned or cut into strips
1 handful or 1 small container cilantro
1 handful or 1 small container fresh basil
2 scallions, greens only cut diagonally

PS 1. Wet a tea towel and wring it out and place it on a board or countertop to roll your rice paper rolls without sticking.
2. Fill a flat casserole pan (large enough to dip the rice paper into) with warm water.
3. Prepare all vegetables and place on a plate separately.
4. Take a piece rice sheet and dampen it with the water for a couple of seconds to soften, but firm. It will continue to soften as you work so work quickly.
5. Place the rice paper on the tea towel and grab some of each of the vegetables and layer into the spring roll. Do not overfill because it will tear the rice paper.
6. Fold top edge down, then side edges in and roll up. Place on parchment paper or a plate until ready to eat. Dip in Thai "Peanut" Sauce (see recipe), or you can layer it in your wrap. Enjoy!

Healing Carrot Tuna

6 carrot sticks, grated (easily done in the high-speed blender under pulse, drain juice, and drink)
1 celery stalk, sliced
½ c sweet onion
¼ dulse flakes
2 tsp tahini
½ lemon juice
½ t ground garlic
salt to taste

PS Combine carrots (drain liquid by mashing into a strainer, or even better, save the pulp after juicing carrots. It is the perfect consistency for tuna), celery, onion, dulse flakes, tahini lemon juice, garlic and salt to taste. Use an ice cream scooper to scoop on top of a large green leaf lettuce or romaine lettuce. You can also make it into a lettuce wrap. The presentation is everything. Enjoy!

Healing Broccoli

fresh broccoli, cut into bite-size pieces

PS Serve with Healing Nacho Cheeze Sauce or Healing Guacamole (see recipe)

Healing Carrot Sticks with Nacho Cheeze Sauce

2-4 carrots cut into sticks or julienned

PS For "cheese sauce (see recipe). Enjoy!

Healing Raw Vegetables (1)

1 c cherry tomatoes
1 cucumber, quartered
1 red pepper, sliced
1 orange pepper, sliced

2-4 leaves of kale, broken into pieces

PS Slice cucumbers and break broccoli florets and cauliflower florets in to bite size pieces. The sweet peppers can be sliced or eaten whole. I like to keep the baby carrots and cherry tomatoes whole. Enjoy!

Healing Raw Vegetables (2)

1 broccoli stalk of florets
1 c organic cherry tomatoes
1 c cauliflower
1 c cucumber, diced
1/2 red bell pepper, sliced
1/2 yellow pepper, sliced
1/2 c baby carrots

PS Slice cucumbers and break broccoli florets and cauliflower florets in to bite size pieces. The sweet peppers can be sliced or eaten whole. I like to keep the baby carrots and cherry tomatoes whole. Enjoy!

Healing Garlic and Basil Salad Dressing

¼ c amino acids
¼ c organic apple cider vinegar with the mother (I prefer Bragg's)
1 T nutritional yeast flakes
1 scallion, sliced (greens only)
1 large garlic clove
1 t onion powder
1 t fresh basil
2 T raw honey

PS As simple as always, put all ingredients except fresh basil and scallions in a high-speed blender and mix well. Toss in chopped basil and scallions.

Healing Ginger-Orange Salad Dressing

1 orange, peeled and seeded
¼ c tamari
1 garlic clove, coarsely chopped
1-inch fresh ginger

12 leaves and stems of fresh cilantro
¼ t orange zest
1 T maple syrup, optional

PS   Place all ingredients in a high-speed blender and blend smooth. Refrigerate or serve immediately. Enjoy!

Healing Sumac Salad Dressing

1 lemon, juiced
2 T honey
1 T amino acid
1 large garlic clove, finely chopped
1 heaping T basil, finely chopped
1 T sumac

PS   Ok, so I won't pretend that I always knew what sumac was, but once I found out, I loved it! It is a spice used in Middle Eastern cuisine. It comes from a flowering plant with fruit. The fruit is dried and ground into a powder and used as a spice. There are over 35 different species. It is usually added to salad and rice dishes and adds such incredible flavor.

I like discovering new and different flavors adding something extra to my regular meals. It excites me. When I added it to this salad dressing, it took it to another level. Not only did it add to the taste, but it is very high in antioxidants, so it added to the nutritional importance during the detoxification process. Knowing this made it even better. When you try it, you will love it too.

You can pick it up at the Indian or Mediterranean markets. It is worth the trip for minimal cost. It is versatile enough to use on any salad. Enjoy!

Healing Mango Dressing

1 mango, chopped
1 garlic clove
½ c apple cider vinegar
¼ c maple syrup
2 T tamari
2 T fresh cilantro, chopped

PS Place all ingredients in a high-speed blender and blend smooth. Serve on your favorite salad. Enjoy!

Healing Cilantro Lime Dressing

2 limes, juiced
1 c fresh cilantro, packed
½ c apple cider vinegar
1 c Bragg's amino acids or tamari
1 garlic clove
¼ c maple syrup
¼ c water

PS Place all ingredients in a high-speed blender and blend smooth. Serve on your favorite salad. Enjoy!

Healing Cilantro Lemon Salad Dressing

20 sprigs cilantro (I don't count them. I grab a handful)
juice of 1 ½ lemon
½ c water
1 clove garlic
1 T maple syrup (optional)
pinch of salt

PS Place all ingredients in a high-speed blender and blend smooth. Add a pinch of salt if desired. Enjoy!

Healing Orange Blossom Salad Dressing

2 T lemon juice
1 garlic clove, finely chopped
½ t coriander seed
1 t orange blossom water
2 t fennel seeds, lightly crushed
juice of 1 orange about 3 T fresh orange juice

PS Put all ingredients in a blender and blend to smoothness. Enjoy!

Healing Beet Salad Dressing

1 T apple cider vinegar (with the mother)
1 T honey
1 T pineapple juice

2 T amino acids or tamari
1 clove garlic, minced
1 T fresh cilantro

PS Mix all ingredients together. This dressing is versatile and can be used on many salads to add zest and flavor. It is recommended to use on the beet salad. Enjoy!

Healing Green Chili Lime Salad Dressing

2 green chilis, seeded and thinly sliced diagonally
2 T lime juice
1 T amino acids
1 T ACV

PS Excellent with Healing Avocado Salad if desired. Enjoy!

Simple Dressing

1 t apple cider vinegar with the mother
1 T Tamari or amino acids
1 garlic clove, coarsely chopped
1 T local honey

PS   Put all ingredients in a magic bullet or blender and blend smooth. Use on any salad you choose for a simple, yet elegant taste. Enjoy!

Notes and Favorites

Sauces
Soups
and Such

Contrary to popular belief, the original diet had nothing to do with hunting or gathering. It had nothing to do with grains or no grains. The original menu was plant food. Genesis 1:29 says "I give you every seed-bearing plant on the face of the whole earth and every tree that has fruit with seed in it. They will be yours for food".

Even animals including lions, elephants, and any even prehistoric animals actively participated in the same type of diet. "And to all the beasts of the earth and all the birds in the sky and all the creatures that move along the ground—everything that has the breath of life in it — I give every green plant for food" (Genesis 1:30). Can you imagine that even animals ate plants? That was their choice of food.

The original diet consisted of plants with seeds in them and also included trees that had fruit on them, which incidentally had and still has seeds in them. That means plants will produce seed or have seed in them. If it has been genetically modified or hybridized, it may lack seeds. Chose a different food.

It is intuitive that the trees and plants at that time were not tainted by all the chemicals we use today. Instead, they were pure and delicious.

We find ourselves reverting to the original diet these days. Why? Because science is finally catching up with the Biblical account of what foods promote healing of the body. Every bite of food you take will either inhibit healing or support it. Chose foods that heal. Choose plants. Eat them deliciously.

Healing Carrot Ginger Soup

3 c baby carrots
2 c fresh kale
1 t onion powder
1 t turmeric
½ t ground cumin
1 T sweet onion
1½ inch ginger
2 T cashews
½ lime juice
salt

PS Put all ingredients in a high-speed blender and blend until smooth. It will heat in the container after about 5 minutes if you have a Vitamix. You will have to mix longer to smooth it if you do not have a high-speed blender. Enjoy!

Healing Portabella Mushroom & Sage Soup

¼ sweet onion
1 large garlic clove
¼ t fennel seeds
1 T sage including the soft stems (remove the woody portions)
1 package baby Bella mushrooms
1 T raw cashews
Add water to your preference
Salt to taste

PS Put all ingredients into a high-speed blender and process about 5 1/2 minutes. I use a Vitamix. It will be hot without being cooked. The food enzymes will be well preserved. Enjoy!

Healing Creamy Tomato Basil Soup

6 medium tomatoes
1 large garlic clove
2 T fresh basil
¼ c raw cashews
1 T oregano
2 T nutritional yeast flakes

PS Wash tomatoes and other vegetables. Maintain skin and seeds of tomatoes. Place all ingredients in a high-speed blender. Blend smooth 5-6 minutes or until nicely warmed. Garnish with fresh basil. Enjoy!

Healing Tomato Carrot Soup

2 medium organic tomatoes, Roma is best
2 carrots, chopped or whole depending on blender
½ avocado
1 large garlic glove
1 t each onion powder
1 t garlic powder

1 t dried oregano
2 T amino acids
2 c hot water

PS Place all ingredients in a high-speed blender and blend until smooth and creamy. In a Vitamix, the soup will be warm. Enjoy!

Healing Tomato Bell Soup

6 Roma tomatoes
1 red bell pepper, seeded
½ avocado, peeled and cored
Juice of ½ lemon
1 small garlic clove, or more to your taste
1 stalk of fresh oregano, leaves only
3 fresh basil leaves
½ t dried basil (gives a peppery flavor)
Himalayan sea salt to taste

PS Blend together tomatoes, pepper, avocado, and garlic. Then add in spices and blend till smooth. Enjoy!

Healing Butternut Squash with Sage and Fennel Soup

1 large butternut squash, diced (about 2 ½ c)
1 fresh garlic clove, minced
1 t onion powder
1 t smoked paprika
¼ t fennel seeds
1 T maple syrup (optional)
2 c warm water (if you prefer a thick consistency add less, thin consistency, add more)
1 t unbleached sea salt, such as pink Himalayan (taste before adding and then add judiciously)
1 sprig fresh sage, with tender part of the stem
extra sage leaf for garnish

PS Blend all the ingredients in a high-speed blender. Carefully add water a little at a time. Blend until smooth. Adjust seasoning as desired. Enjoy!

Healing Coconut Soup

1 young coconut, fresh or frozen

1 medium tomato
1-inch fresh galangal or fresh ginger
3 cloves fresh garlic
Juice of 1 fresh lime or ½ lemon
1 t curry powder
½ t red pepper flakes
¼ t salt
2 T fresh cilantro.
¼ c   bean sprouts or mung beans
¼ c scallions, sliced on the diagonal, green parts only

PS Open a young coconut. It is not easy, but it is not impossible. People cut them all the time. Remove the husk from the top of the coconut so that there are no strings attached when you pop open the top.

In Thailand, they cut a "u" shape in the point of the coconut with a large sharp knife being careful to cut away from the body. Place it on a firm surface before cutting. It takes a bit of force and a sharp knife to cut at a 45° angle through the hard shell. Use the edge of the blade to pop open the top. Pour off the water into a high-speed blender and scrape out the meat and place into the blender.

Add garlic, galangal (or ginger), tomato, curry powder, lime juice, chili flakes, and salt. Blend until smooth. Divide sprouts between 2 dishes. Pour soup mixture into the bowl and garnish with cilantro and scallions. Enjoy!

Healing Guacamole

2 ripe avocados
½ c red onions, chopped
½ fresh cilantro, chopped
1 garlic clove, minced
1 t onion powder
½ - 1 t smoked paprika
Juice of 1 lime
pinch of salt

PS Mash avocado in a bowl. Add the rest of the ingredients saving the lime juice and mix thoroughly. Squeeze in fresh lime juice. Use with raw vegetables. Enjoy!

Healing Thai "Peanut" Sauce

½ c fresh almonds
1 garlic clove, minced
1 T fresh ginger, grated
¼ c amino acids
¼ c apple cider vinegar
1 T honey or maple syrup
¼ c fresh lime
¼ c water

PS In high-speed blender, pulse almonds to a flour consistency. Add lime juice, garlic, ginger, honey, amino acids, and apple cider vinegar in a blender and blend smooth. Use water to thin if necessary. Stir in red pepper flakes. Serve with Asian wraps or salads.

Healing Nacho "Cheese" Sauce

3½ c water for soaking cashews

2 c raw cashews, soaked cashews

1 T nutritional yeast flakes

1 t salt

1 t ground garlic

1 garlic clove

juice of ½ lime

1 T apple cider vinegar

1 t cayenne pepper

1 t hot smoked paprika (can use mild if desired)

1 c water

¼ c chopped red pepper

PS Soak cashews in filtered water for 2-3 hours then drain. Place soaked cashews in a high-speed blender. Add the other ingredients except for salt. Add salt slowly and taste as to not over salt the sauce. Blend until smooth. The sauce may be used in casseroles, as a cheese dip, in Mexican dishes or placed in a dehydrator until firm. Your choice.

Healing Cheeze

2 c raw cashews

1½ c water

½ red bell pepper, coarsely chopped

juice of 1 lemon

3 T nutritional yeast flakes

1 T tahini (exclude oil)

1 clove garlic

1 t smoked paprika

1 t granulated onion powder

1 t salt

PS This is incredibly easy to make. The longest part is waiting for it to dehydrate, which takes about 24 hours. I make it up sometimes after work. Just put all ingredients into the high-speed blender and blend until smooth and creamy. Spread onto parchment lined dehydrator trays (I use 2) and dehydrate at 110° for about 12 hours or overnight. Flip it over and remove parchment paper and dehydrate 8-12 hours longer depending on your desired texture. The longer it is dehydrated, the crispier it gets. I like mine to be the consistency of cheese slices. I made it with onion bread, and it was unexpectedly delicious. Enjoy!

Healing Onion Bread

1 large sweet onion, sliced in rings
¾ c ground sunflowers
¾ c ground flaxseeds
¼ c amino acids
¼ c water
1 T nutritional yeast flakes, optional
1 t smoked paprika
1 t ground onion powder
1 apple, pureed
2 sprigs of fresh rosemary, tender leaves only

PS Place all dry ingredients in a large bowl, combine well. Add amino acids and water and stir well. In a blender, puree an apple and add 2 sprigs of fresh rosemary. Add to mixture. Fold in ringed onions and mix well. Allow the batter to rest about 30 minutes to soften the onions. Spread the mixture onto parchment paper or Teflex to a thickness of about ⅛ - ¼ inch.

Dehydrate for 12 hours at 110° or until the surface is no longer sticky. Flip bread and remove parchment paper and continue to dehydrate until firm and dry or to your desired consistency. Anywhere from 8-24 hours.

Cool to room temperature and cut to preferred size and shape. Onion bread may be stored in a glass container in a cool, dry place for up to 6 months, but it will be eaten way before then. Mine only lasted a few days. Enjoy!

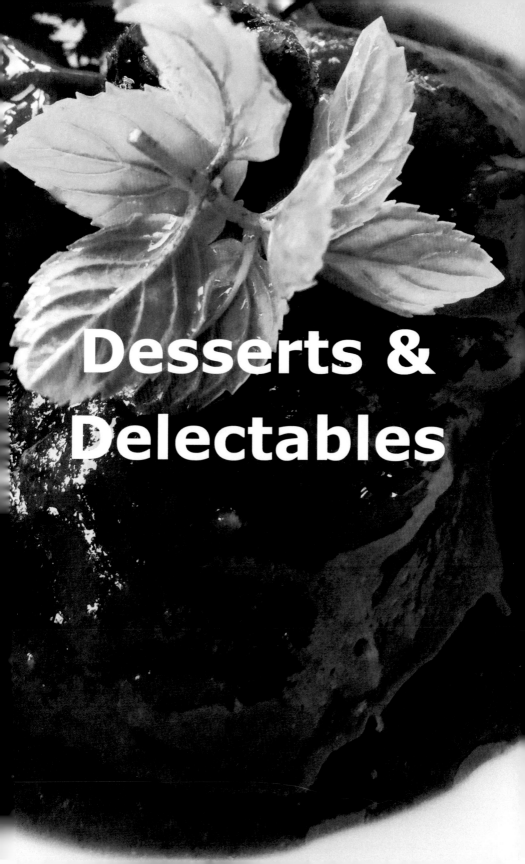

Desserts & Delectables

Everyone loves sweets. The delectables recorded here are made with safe ingredients. The great thing about it is that no one has to know they are healthy unless you tell them. Shh!

Healing Almond Butter Apple Sandwich

2 pink lady apples
1-2 T natural almond butter

PS Slice apples in rounds. Spread almond butter on one side of the slice and place a second slice on top to form a sandwich. Enjoy!

Walnuts

½ c raw walnuts, best soaked overnight, drained and dehydrated.

PS Pour desired amount of walnuts into a bowl and cover with water. Leave overnight. In the morning, drain and rinse walnuts. Place on dehydrator tray in a single layer and dehydrate about 24 hours.   I want them to be thoroughly dry so that they will last longer.

The purpose of soaking the walnuts is to remove the enzyme inhibitor from nuts for better digestion.

Almonds and Blueberries

1 pint organic blueberries
1 handful of almonds, soaked and dehydrated if available

PS Blueberries are a very high antioxidant fruit. I particularly like them for their anti-aging effect. I eat them all the time and in large amounts. Sometimes I have it in the morning because I use them for breakfast. I munch on them until lunchtime between seeing patients.

The protein from the almonds give it lasting power and holds me until lunch time. The mixture of berries and almonds is an excellent combination for detoxification and rejuvenation. The berries are sweet, and the almonds are delicious and crunchy. Together, or even individually, it is a great snack. Enjoy!

Healing Anti-Aging Berries

1 pint blackberries
1 pint raspberries
1 pint blueberries

PS Mix berries together and use as a relaxing snack or anytime. Enjoy!

Healing Cherries

Fresh Organic Cherries, 1-2 cups

PS   Cherries are a great antioxidant food that helps to scavenge the free radicals that want to damage your cells and cause disease. Why not stop a disease from running rampant in your body with a nice bowl of cherries red or Ranier. They are also a great sleep aid. Enjoy!

Healing Rawlicious Granola

1 cup almonds, chopped, soaked and dehydrated if available
2 T ground flaxseed
⅓ c sunflower seeds
⅓ c pumpkin seeds
⅓ c raisins
⅓ c dried, chopped apples
⅓ c local honey or maple syrup
2 T water
1 t vanilla extract
1 t cinnamon
⅛ t nutmeg
¼ t Himalayan salt

PS Mix all the dry ingredients in a large bowl. Whisk together the honey, water, cinnamon, nutmeg, vanilla, and salt. Pour over dry ingredients and mix them well with your hands. Spread out evenly on parchment paper on dehydrator racks. Dehydrate at 115 degrees for about 10-12 hours, or until granola is sticky but adhering firmly. Refrigerate till ready eat to maintain crunchiness.

Healing Strawberry Nice Cream

2 c raw cashew, soaked about 1 hour
1 c fresh or frozen young coconut meat
8 oz fresh strawberries
1 c coconut water
4-6 Medjool dates, soaked in warm water to soften and pitted
1 full vanilla bean or 1 t vanilla extract
Juice of 1 lemon
Pinch of Himalayan salt

PS Drain the soaked cashews and dates and rinse cashews. Add all ingredients to a high-speed blender and blend until smooth and creamy. At this point, you have two options. The first is to refrigerate for an hour and then use ice cream maker to churn. Transfer to steel loaf pan and freeze overnight or about 8 hours. The second is to transfer mixture directly into steel loaf pan and freeze overnight until firm. Enjoy!

Healing Cherry Sorbet

4 c frozen organic cherries
1 lime, juiced
1 T water
2 Medjool dates (optional)

PS In a high-speed blender, blend soaked dates (if using) and water with lime to break the wall of the dates. Add cherries and process until well combined, and into a mound. Garnish with fresh mint. I use a Vitamix, and it makes fabulous sorbet and ice creams. Dates are optional, but should be soaked in hot water for about 10 minutes to soften. If you would like the sorbet firmer, freezes for 2 hours and then eat. Enjoy!

Healing Pineapple Ginger Sorbet

1 fresh pineapple, cut into 2-inch pieces
3 inches of fresh ginger, peeled
2 T fresh lemon juice
raspberries for garnish

PS Place pineapple, ginger and lemon juice in a food processor or high-speed blender and process until smooth. Pour mixture into an ice cream maker and follow instructions or spoon into a glass bowl with tight lid. Freeze for 3 hours until it is hard on the outside and soft on the inside.

Remove the container from the freezer and whisk until smooth then return to the freezer for another 4 hours or until firm. Garnish with raspberries for taste and color. Enjoy!

Healing Ice Greens

3 c kale, stems removed
3 c spinach
½ c almonds
1 c water
2 bananas
½ avocado
2 T lemon juice
2 T almond extract
1 c sliced or whole raw almonds to garnish (optional)
2-4 Medjool dates, optional
pinch of salt
3 c ice

This is an easy "ice cream" make. Don't let the name fool you. Put all ingredients into a high blender and blend well. For consistent results, use an ice cream maker. If you don't have an ice cream maker, place the ice green in a shallow bowl in the freezer and stir every 30 minutes. To harden the ice green, freeze it for 1-2 hours. If the ice green is in the freezer for a few days, you will need to thaw it 15-30 minutes to allow it to soften. Enjoy!

Healing Nutty Granola

1 c soaked and dehydrated pecans
1 c soaked and dehydrated almonds
1 c pumpkin seeds
1 c goji berries or other dried fruit
2 apples (see below)
3-5 dates, pitted and soaked in water (to 1 c total water and dates, save water)
1 t cinnamon
1 t vanilla extract
1 t butterscotch or almond extract
1 t salt

PS Pulse pecans and almonds in a blender to leave small chunks. Remove. Mix in pumpkin seeds and goji berries. At this point, the nuts can be seasoned with cinnamon, extracts, and salt and eaten.

Alternatively, place in a dehydrator for granola that can be broken into pieces or cut into bars. Here's how: In the same high-speed blender, process apples, dates, cinnamon, vanilla, butterscotch and salt into applesauce. Toss into nut mixture. Spread on dehydrator tray layered with unbleached parchment paper. Dehydrate at 105° overnight or at least 8-10 hours. Break into pieces by hand or cut into bars.

Healing Apple Cinnamon Cashew Cookies

2 c raw cashews
1 apple, cored, quartered (leave the skin on)
1 T flaxseeds
2 t cinnamon
1 t salt
1 c raw cashews, folded in
¼ c chopped figs
¼ c water

PS Grind cashews and flaxseeds to a flour consistency in the high-speed blender. Add apple, cinnamon and salt. Next add water. The mixture will be gooey. Fold in cashews and raisins. Dehydrate 15 hours for a firm outside and gooey inside or eat them without dehydration. Just refrigerate for 1-2 hours for firmness. Enjoy!

Healing Lemon Rosemary Cookies

4 c raw almonds
2 lemons, peeled and cut lengthwise to expel the seeds
3 t vanilla extract
3 T fresh rosemary
4-6 dates, soaked 10 minutes
1 t salt

PS Place almonds in a high-speed blender and use the damper to mix in the nuts. If you are using a Vitamix, start on low speed and then increase to 8. If it overheats, turn it off a few minutes and restart. If you are not using a high-speed blender, blend longer. You may require a little water to get the almonds going.

Once the mixture becomes moistened (about 5-10 minutes depending on the stopping time) add lemon, rosemary, dates, vanilla, and salt. Combine well. It will make a nice moistened cookie dough. Roll in in 2 inch balls and then flatten on a cookie sheet and refrigerate for 2 hours. Enjoy!

A second option is to use a dehydrator and dehydrate the cookies for 2 hours or until desired consistency. The longer you dehydrate the cookies, the crispier they will become.

Healing Avocado Nice Dream

1 avocado
2 c coconut milk
½ cup organic tahini (sesame seed paste)
1 cup maple syrup or your favorite sweetener
¼ teaspoon salt
1 t vanilla extract
2 T fresh basil, chopped
2 T fresh lemon juice
2 cups strawberries, maintain tops

PS Blend milk, maple syrup, tahini, avocado, salt and vanilla in your blender. Blend until creamy and place in your ice-cream maker. In a separate container, pulse strawberries, lemon and basil and then combine with milk mixture. Place in ice cream maker and proceed according to package instructions. Store ice cream in an airtight container. Enjoy!

Sample Meal Plans and Shopping Lists

Reverse It Sample Meal Plan

Meal plan for the week

	7am	9:30 am	12 noon	2:30 pm	5pm	7:30pm
Sunday	Get Me Started!	The Beet Goes On or Roman Beet	Partial to Parsley or The Greenery	Kale-Aboration	Vision	Gingered Lemon Shot
Monday	The Eye Opener	Red Runner	The Greenery	Bringing In The Greens	I'm Kale'n It	C-Shot
Tuesday	Vision	Anti-Flam	Roman Beet	I'm Kale'n It	The Beet Goes On	Shot to Kill
Wednesday	Roman Beet	Allergy Bust Shot	Kale-Aboration	Ridiculous	Keep It Movin' Shot	Green Beet
Thursday	The Beet Goes On	Italian Sipper	The Eye Opener	Bringing In The Greens	Kick Some Kale	Heavy Metal Buster Shot
Friday	Get Me Started!	Shot To Kill	Anti-Flam	Vision	Kale-Aboration	Puttin Out The Fire
Saturday	Kick Some Kale	Red Runner	The Greenery	Partial To Parsley	C-Shot	Red Runner

*This is intended to provide examples only. You will be able to mix and match to allow it to fit into your lifestyle. Remember to squeeze 1/2 lemon into 16 0z of room temperature purified or alkaline water upon awakening. Drink 16 oz of purified or alkaline water in between "meals". Try drinking water 30 minutes prior to your "meal" or 30 minutes after your "meal". Plant-based raw foods have enzymes in them requiring your body to do less to digest the foods while allowing your body the opportunity to heal. The most difficult days are days 3-5. Hang in there! Use body products without parabens, phthalates or pore clogging elements. Try Our Body Detox Line that includes Detox Shower Gel, Detox Body Lotion, Detox Body Scrub and Detox Body Deodorant. See www.pain2wellness healthcare.com for more details. If detox symptoms occur, try vegetable broth and then restart.

#1 Sample Juice Menu

Healing Sample Meal Plan

Meal plan for the week

	Breakfast	Snack 1	Lunch	Snack 2	Dinner
Sunday	Healing Pineapple Tangerine Cream Smoothie	Healing Anti-Aging Berries	Healing Pineapple Beet Salad	Healing Anti-Aging Berries/Handful of Almonds(≈15 almonds)	Healing Give It a Rest Smoothie
Monday	Italian Sipper	Healing Onion Bread with Healing Guacamole	Healing Carrot Tuna with Green Leaf or Romain Lettuce	Healing Citrus Bowl	Healing Carrot Ginger Soup and Choice of Salad
Tuesday	Healing Pitaya Bowl	Healing Lemon Rosemary Cookies	Healing Coconut Soup with Healing Asian Wraps with Thai "Peanut" Sauce	Healing Onion Bread with Healing Cheeze	Healing Tomato Bell Soup with Healing Mixed Greens Salad and Onion Bread
Wednesday	Healing Blueberry Beat Smoothie	Healing Almond Butter Apple Sandwich	Healing Portabella Mushroom and Sage Soup	Healing Broccoli with Nacho Cheeze Sauce	Healing Parental Discretion Advisement Smoothie
Thursday	The Eye Opener	Healing Nutty Granola	Healing All In Salad	Healing Carrot Sticks with Healing Guacamole	Healing Vegetable Korma
Friday	Healing Tropical C Smoothie	Healing Fruit Casserole	Healing Corn and Kale Salad	Healing Pineapple Tangerine Cream Smoothie	Healing Kale in Coconut Wrap with Healing Strawberry Nice Cream
Saturday	Healing Overnight Oats	Healing Beet Salad	Healing Pineapple Beet Salad	Healing Raw Vegetables with Cheeze Sauce or Guacamole	Healing Curry Chick'n Salad In Collard Wrap

*This is intended to provide examples only. You will be able to mix and match to allow it to fit into your lifestyle. Remember to squeeze 1/2 lemon into 16 0z of room temperature purified or alkaline water upon awakening. Drink 16 oz of purified or alkaline water in between "meals". Try drinking water 30 minutes prior to your "meal" or 30 minutes after your "meal". Plant-based raw foods have enzymes in them requiring your body to do less to digest the foods while allowing your body the opportunity to heal. The most difficult days are days 3-5. Hang in there! Use body products without parabens, phthalates or pore clogging elements. Try Our Body Detox Line that includes Detox Shower Gel, Detox Body Lotion, Detox Body Scrub and Detox Body Deodorant. See www.pain2wellness healthcare.com for more details. If detox symptoms occur; try vegetable broth and then restart. Peanuts are not used due to the aflatoxins. Almonds make a great substitution. If allergic, please omit.

#2 Sample Healing Menu

A Day In the Life Juicing Menu

Shopping List

Item	Qty	Fresh Food Store
Spinach large clamshells	2	
Kale	2	
Fennel bulb and stems	1	
Parsley	1	
Mint	1	
Celery	4	
Cucumbers	5	
Green Apple	1	
Limes	3	
Pears	3	
Carrots	16	
Romaine Head	2	
Beet large	1	
Ginger	1	
Oranges	7	
Lemon	1	
Tangerines	6	

#3 "A Day In The Life" Sample Juice Shopping List, Sunday

184

A Day In the Life Healing Menu

Shopping List

Item	Qty	Fresh Food Store
Kale	10 c	
Avocado	1	
Chia seeds	1 c	
Frozen Blueberries	1 c	
Lavender petals or tea petals	1 t	
Lemon	1	
Almonds	15	
Pineapple	1 1/4 c	
Beet large	1	
Ginger	1	
Local honey	1	
Tangerines	3	
Pine Nuts	2 T	
Fresh berries (blueberries/ raspberries/strawberries/blackberries	1 each	

c= cups, t=teaspoon, T=tablespoon

#4   "A Day In The Life"   Sample Healing Shopping List
Sunday

Make Your Own Shopping List

Shopping List

Item	Qty	Fresh Food Store

c= cups, t=teaspoon, T=tablespoon

#5   "A Day In The Life"   Make Your Own Shopping List

Conclusion

The Standard American Diet (SAD) revolves around processed foods with empty calories. There are too many "toos"--too much salt, too much sugar, too much of the wrong protein and too little health-promoting foods. This has lead to obesity, heart disease, diabetes and many forms of cancer. The increasing number of sick people is staggering and the number continues to climb.

There is overwhelming scientific evidence that reveals the secret of optimal health. Just a few of the benefits include

1. Improved immunity,

2. Better digestion,

3. Decreased cancer risk,

4. Reversal of chronic conditions such as heart disease and type 2 diabetes,

5. Prevention and reversal of erectile dysfunction,

6. Decreased blood pressure,

7. Promotion of effortless weight loss,

8. Promotion of younger, vibrant skin,

9. Promotion of longevity,

10. Increased energy,

11. Improved sleep,

12. Improved mood,

13. Increased mental clarity and,

14. Decreased need for many medications.

This list of benefits is by no means exhaustive, but it is significant.

Food satisfies hunger, but more importantly, it provides the fuel that keeps our bodies healthy and robust. The body can function on suboptimal fuel for some time, but it will do so at a cost. Once the body's reserves are compromised, the debt increases.

People often complain about the cost of healthful living, but you will pay for it one way or another. To have robust and lasting health, the body must have the right fuel. It is better to pay the fuel cost upfront instead of paying it on the backend. The cost of disease is much higher.

Hippocrates, the father of medicine, said in 400 BC "Let Food Be Thy Medicine and Medicine Thy Food." He knew the importance of food way back then. Since his time, many scientific studies have documented food's medicinal properties and how our food choices can prevent disease or promote it.

We have too long been stalled by the status quo of "business as usual" with type 2 diabetes. Check your blood sugar. Use this medicine. Amputate this leg. It is overwhelming.

The collateral damage of type 2 diabetes including cardiovascular disease, hypercholesterolemia, hypertension, kidney failure, amputations, peripheral neuropathy, Alzheimers and others has to be enough to want to rise up and take control to promote health and reverse type 2 diabetes through scientifically proven alternatives.

Many of the Hollywood stars take full advantage of the benefits of proper foods and the use of appropriate detoxification for health, beauty, and wellness. We know that the proper foods reverse chronic diseases and are meant for more than just beauty.

Hollywood benefits from healthy foods and how they improve health, beauty, and wellness. Now you can benefit too.

Type 2 diabetes is only a challenge. It is like a boxing match, like the boxing challenge of Creed. He overcame his challenge victoriously. He had the tools.

Now you have the tools to fight your challenge. You can overcome your challenge victoriously. Put your gloves on and go for it! We have provided you with your best punch. Put your gloves on and give it your best shot. Give the old one two. **Reverse it!**

References

1. Becoming Raw, Brenda Davis, R.D., Vesanto Melina, MS, R.D., Ryan Berry, Book Publishing Company, 2010.

2. Rohrmann, S. Meat and Dairy Consumption and the Subsequent Cancer in a US Cohort Study. Cancer Causes Control 2007; 18:41-50.

3. Campbell, T., & Campbell, T. (2005). The China Study: Startling Implications For Diet, Weight Loss and Long-Term Health, The Most Comprehensive Study of Nutrition Ever Conducted. BenBella Books, 2005.

4. Centers for Disease Control and Prevention. Diabetes Basics, A National Epidemic, 2017; http://cdc.gov.

5. World Health Organization. Home/News/ Fact sheets/Detail/Diabetes, 2018; http://who.int.

6. Diabetes, I. M. Stratton, A. L. Adler, and H.A. Neil, "Association of Glycaemia with Macrovascular and Microvascular Complications of Type 2 Diabetes (UKPDS 35): Prospective Observational Study," British Medical Journal 321 (2000): 405-12.

7. American Diabetes Association. Our Mission. 1995-2018; http://diabetes.org.

8. J.R.W Brownrigg, J. Apelqvist, K. Bakker, N.C. Schaper, and R. J. Hinchliffe. Evidence-based managed of PAD & the Diabetic Foot. European Journal of Vascular and Endovasular Surgery,

2013. 45(6): p. 673-681. http://www.ejves.com/
article/S1078-5884 (13)00136-6/abstract
(accessed 12/1/2018).

9. M. A. Shammas, Telomeres, lifestyle, cancer and
    aging. Current Opinion in Clinical Nutrition and
    Metabolic Care. 2011 Jan; 14(1):28-34.

10. A.S. Nicholson et al., "Toward Improved
    Management of NIDDM: A Randomized ,
    Controlled , Pilot Intervention Using a Low-Fat,
    Vegetarian Diet," Preventive Medicine 29 (1999):
    87-91.

11. N. D. Barnard et al., "The Effects of a Low-Fat,
    Plant-Based Dietary Intervention on Body Weight,
    Metabolism, and Insulin Sensitivity." American
    Journal of Medicine 118 (2005): 991-7.

12. Health Power, Hans Diehl, Dr.HSc. , MPH, /Aileen
    Ludington, MD, Review and Herald Publishing
    Association, 2016.

13. Goodbye Lupus, by Brooke Goldner, MD, Express
    Results, LLC, 2015.

14. Prevent and Reverse Heart Disease, by Caldwell
    B. Esselstyn, Jr., MD, The Penguin Group, 2008.

15. D. Ornish et al., "Intensive Lifestyle Changes for
    Reversal of Coronary Heart Disease," Journal of
    the American Medical Association 280 (1998)
    2001-7.

16. A. V. Greco et al, "Insulin Resistance in Morbid
    Obesity: reversal with Intramyocellular Fat
    Depletion," Diabetes 52 (2002): 144-51.

17. L. M. Goff et al.,Veganism and Its Relationship with Insulin Resistance and Intramyocellular Lipid," European Journal of Clinical Nutrition 59 (2005): 291-8.

18. Dr. Neal Barnard's program for Reversing Diabetes. The Scientifically Proven System for Reversing Diabetes Without Drugs, Neal D. Barnard, MD, Rodale Inc. 2007.

19. The Simple Way to Lose Weight and Reverse Illness, Using The China Study's Whole-Food, Plant-Based Diet, by Thomas Campbell, MD, Rodale Inc. 2015.

20. Reversing Diabetes, Reduce or Even Eliminate Your Dependence on Insulin or Oral Drugs, by Julian Whitaker, MD. Hachette Book Group, 1990

21. N Chalasani, et al, "The diagnosis and management of nonalcoholic fatty liver disease: Practice guidance from the American Association for the Study of Liver Diseases" . Hepatology. 67 (1) (2018):328-357.

22. Non-alcoholic fatty liver disease (NAFLD): assessment and management/Guidance and guidelines. NICE. July 2016. J. Glen, et al (September 2016). "Non-alcoholic fatty liver disease: summary of NICE guidance" . BMJ. 354: i4428.

23. H. Tilt, A.R. Moschen, M. Roden, "NALFD and Diabetes Mellitus" . Nature Reviews. Gastroenterology & Hepatology. 14 (1)(2017): 32-42.

24. Rudd's-Clausen, C.F. et al. Olive, Soybean and Palm Oils Intake Have a Similar Acute Detrimental Effect Over the Endothelial Function in Healthy Young Subjects. Nutrition, Metabolism & Cardiovascular Diseases 2007; 17 (1): 50-7.

25. McGarry J.D: Banting Lecture 2001: Deregulation of Fatty Acid Metabolism in the Etiology of Type 2 Diabetes. Diabetes 51 : 7-18, 2002.

26. Randle P.J., Garland P.B., Hales C.N. Newsholme E.A.: The Glucose Fatty-Acid Cycle. It's Roll in Insulin Sensitivity and the Metabolic Disturbances of Diabetes Mellitus. Lancet 1 : 785-789, 1963.

27. Sparks, L. M., Xie, H., Mynatt, R., Hulver, M.W., Bray, G.A., Smith, S.R.: A High-Fat Diet Coordinately Downregulates Genes Required for Mitochondrial Oxidative Phosphorylation In Skeletal Muscle. Diabetes 54(7), 1923-1933, 2005.